Public Health
in Appalachia

CONTRIBUTIONS TO SOUTHERN APPALACHIAN STUDIES

Public Health in Appalachia

Essays from the Clinic and the Field

Edited by WENDY WELCH

Foreword by John Dreyzehner

CONTRIBUTIONS TO SOUTHERN APPALACHIAN STUDIES, 35

McFarland & Company, Inc., Publishers
Jefferson, North Carolina

"When OxyContin Struck, and How the Community Struck Back: One Woman Remembers" by Sue Ella Kobak is revised from *Transforming Places: Lessons from Appalachia,* edited by Stephen L. Fisher and Barbara Ellen Smith. Copyright 2012 by the Board of Trustees of the University of Illinois. Used with the permission of the University of Illinois Press.

LIBRARY OF CONGRESS CATALOGUING-IN-PUBLICATION DATA

Public health in Appalachia : essays from the clinic and the field /
    edited by Wendy Welch ; foreword by John Dreyzehner.
        p.   cm. — (Contributions to southern Appalachian studies ; 35)
    Includes bibliographical references and index.

    ISBN 978-0-7864-9414-9 (softcover : acid free paper) ∞
    ISBN 978-1-4766-1603-2 (ebook)

    I. Welch, Wendy, editor. II. Series: Contributions to southern
Appalachian studies ; 35.
    [DNLM: 1. Medically Underserved Area—Appalachian Region—
Essays.   2. Health Services Accessibility—Appalachian Region—
Essays.   3. Socioeconomic Factors—Appalachian Region—Essays.
W 76 AA6]
    RA771.6.M37 2014
    362.10974—dc23   2014016720

BRITISH LIBRARY CATALOGUING DATA ARE AVAILABLE

Front cover images © 2014 iStock and Stockbyte

Printed in the United States of America

McFarland & Company, Inc., Publishers
   Box 611, Jefferson, North Carolina 28640
   www.mcfarlandpub.com

Table of Contents

Part Three: Cultural Theory and Clinical Policy

Foreword

Many years ago, a young college student from Chicago signed up for a brief Catholic mission experience deep in rural Appalachia. One of the first things the ignorant young man noticed was that the locals and the host clergy didn't pronounce "Appalachia" right. What they said sounded more like "apple-AT-cha." Fortunately he did not try to correct them, nor they, more kindly, he in saying "app-a-LAY-cha." That was the beginning of an education in cultural sensitivity and cultural literacy. There was a lot to learn.

The second thing that stuck for decades was an hour the young student spent visiting with a very old-appearing, edentulous, and seemingly very lonely man at a local nursing facility. There was little two-way conversation. The nursing home–bound man seemed glad for the company, but through infirmity was not able to express himself meaningfully — until just as it was time for the student to leave. As he stood to say his farewell, the older man reached out to him, taking hold of his arm and suddenly beginning to muster strained sounds, from deep inside himself. He seemed to push the words out of his mouth against a heavy weight that he was determined to move.

"We've all got to work together!" he said, slowly and strained, but with clear conviction. That was it. A gift. A lifetime of wisdom he managed to share with a young man he would never see again. The young man never forgot it. Years later that young man, a bit older, found himself again in Appalachia, trying — not always successfully — to live by that advice.

It is not as easy as all that to "work together." Even when the needs are obvious, the rewards significant and there are few other options, the "We-s" don't always triumph over the "I-s." But most of the meaningful progress in prosperity and health occurs when they do — bringing, ultimately, happiness and the possibility of the fulfillment of human potential, something Appalachia is blessed with an abundance of.

1

The pages of this book detail some of the great strengths, weaknesses, opportunities and threats to this abundance, and to making progress together in Appalachia. And progress has indeed been made — wonderfully so in many places — against the backdrop of a rich rural landscape and a culture that has deeply influenced the nation through more than its share of setbacks, conflict and, indeed, devastation, in its 400-year post–European settlement history. Yes, it is plain Appalachia sees hunger, poverty, health disparities, disability, preventable illness and premature death in too high numbers. A vision to work for the *"continuous improvement in the health and prosperity of the region,"* as the Southwest Virginia Health Authority articulated a few years ago, is necessary to change this. Yet, Appalachia also knows a quiet strength, built on people working together and striving to lift one another up as part of a community and region. In nurturing that, the vision can be realized.

A theme emerges in the health and related essays that follow. Lives can be bettered and progress made when people work together with creativity, passion and innovation — an entrepreneurial spirit of shared ownership in an endeavor as part of a community and a region that provides its own inspiration and reward. I commend these pages to you. Let them speak and weave a picture of a region that has known great adversity, but also great strength. Let the "We–s" have it, and let's all work together, because in Appalachia we must. In Appalachia, we learn it is truly better to serve in heaven, than to reign in that other place.

John Dreyzehner, commissioner of the Tennessee Department of Health, spent nearly fifteen years practicing medicine and raising his family in central Appalachia. For most of that time he was the director of a multi-county health district in far southwest Virginia. He began his health career as an Air Force flight surgeon.

Introduction

This book was conceived under the auspices of the Graduate Medical Education Consortium of Southwest Virginia, an organization tasked with recruiting, retaining, and homegrowing health professionals to work in a rural area of Coalfields Appalachia. It owes much to the then-director of the Consortium, Dr. Gary Crum. Gary retired in 2011 as the executive director, leaving behind an interesting challenge and many wise insights. One of these was that building a health infrastructure with, for, and of the people it served was the most sustainable of all models in an underserved region. Another was that health, education, and economic development are a three-legged stool; any one leg off balance created instability, and led to unsustainability.

What follows here are three segments of an examination along that theme: a section on issues critical to both clinics and communities in Appalachia; a second on potential solutions toward solving long-running healthcare delivery barriers in an underserved region; and a third on theoretical perspectives that can affect policies and delivery of healthcare in Appalachia's diverse regions.

Defining Appalachia is in itself problematic, and the essays in this book reflect the diversity of opinions on the subject. The Appalachian Regional Commission (ARC) defines Appalachia as "a 205,000-square-mile region that follows the spine of the Appalachian Mountains from southern New York to northern Mississippi. It includes all of West Virginia and parts of 12 other states: Alabama, Georgia, Kentucky, Maryland, Mississippi, New York, North Carolina, Ohio, Pennsylvania, South Carolina, Tennessee, and Virginia" (arc.gov). While the ARC's definition is taken as foundational, where and how other areas are considered rural, urban, and underserved is more fluid. Also, the health disparities that abound in Appalachia — high rates of cancer and diabetes, as well as the more subtle assumptions about who the Appalachian people are (or if such a distinct group even exists) — are not standardized between authors. The richness of opinion and the internal voices of the authors provide a rich tapestry of Appalachia's complex and multi-voiced story. As Nigerian novelist Chimamanda Ngozi Adichie has observed, "The single story creates stereotypes, and the problem with stereotypes is not that they are untrue, but that they are incomplete. They make one story become the only story."

Part One of this book, "Health Issues," features some recurring problems rural areas face: dental care, cancer, diabetes, and substance abuse. While none are specific to Appalachia, each presents unique challenges as a result of being in the region. The challenge for those working with these issues is to identify causes that do not blame the victim, that take into account cultural (from lifestyle to geography) specifics of the area, and that seek solutions based on existing regional resources, including plausible funding. The ultimate goal is to posit solutions that are sustainable and effective.

In order to be both (or either) sustainable and effective, those solutions must involve local wisdom and cultural awareness. They must also incorporate long-term development of a medical and economic infrastructure in Appalachia's rural communities, alongside appreciation of the region's intellectual resources in both rural and urban areas. Perhaps the most significant barrier to this ultimate goal includes stereotypes held so long they have become unexamined suppositions. Some of the essays in this section conflict with one another in their positions on common tropes such as fatalism, the role of family, the power of individual choices, and the reasons for economic and educational underachievement in Appalachia, particularly in its rural locations. The purpose of these essays is less definitive answers on age-old problems, than to point out that perhaps the problems carry inside them evolving issues and presumptive beliefs that require re-examining when brought together.

Sarah Raskin and A. Carole Pratt start off with one of the most pervasive and least understood needs: dental care. Jokes about missing teeth are a staple of Appalachian stereotypes. In their work focusing on rural areas, Raskin and Pratt delve deeper and find true pain. Their article pushes past stereotypes to causes: lack of infrastructure, long-term neglect, inadequate funding. And then it pushes forward, to internal solutions within the communities affected, including the building of a rural dental school as an alternate to mobile and free clinics, perhaps as a model for twenty-first century dental practice in America.

Next, Morgan Fields, Gretchen E. Ely and Mark Dignan ask why Appalachia appears to have a higher burden of cancer than other regions of the United States. Is it tobacco culture, industrial pollution, lack of access to health care, under-insurance? All of the above, perhaps? While no one knows the definitive causes, programs to intervene have historically not performed well, and individual behaviors have become the scapegoat for why a problem can't be solved. As cancer trials in Appalachia continue to seek community involvement, they are also beginning to involve community perspective and wisdom. Perhaps this will help change the cancer burden in coalfields Appalachia. Dignan and his team at the University of Kentucky think so, and have worked for many years to involve local wisdom and community knowledge in the larger picture of how to educate on individual behavior while taking into account the many other significant factors at work in areas overburdened with cancer.

Following on from cancer, Carl J. Greever, Rachel Ward and Christian L. Williams examine diabetes. A growing problem across the United States and the world, diabetes rates in Appalachia are significant, while its specific causes in the region are commingled and indeterminate. The authors dissect the medical, behavioral, and environmental anatomy of this chronic disease and apply that foundation to the special circumstances found in Appalachia. Examining the national evolution of dietary changes related to processed foods and high fructose corn syrup (HFCS), the relationships between diabetes and tobacco use, and the twined roles of poverty and educational attainment, they discuss the strengths as well as the weaknesses of the region in a culturally-sensitive context. Noting that this persistent chronic disease problem has no easy fixes no matter where it is found, the authors conclude their analysis with a cogent discussion of some appropriate paths toward the reduction of diabetes prevalence in the face of Appalachia's specific challenges.

Finally, Sue Ella Kobak tackles the thorny issue of substance abuse. In counterpoint to Greever et al.'s focus on patient responsibility, Kobak takes a hard look at corporate responsibility, asking what governance should be in place to keep a mindful eye on the relationships between pill providers, prescribers, and patients. She examines marketing practice, regional cultural attributes, how different states reacted to or even sought to prevent prescriptive painkiller addiction, and the role of the community in safeguarding its own health.

In Part Two, "Culturally Appropriate Healthcare Delivery Systems," contributors examine three different potential models. It has long been a tenet of best business practice that one finds a need and fills it, receiving due financial reward for doing so. Build a better mousetrap — or in this case, a more efficient healthcare delivery system — and the world will beat a path to your door. But when it comes to Appalachia, myriad potential methods for delivering health care exist, while the path is full of hairpin turns and given to icing in winter.

The problems begin when generally recognized best practice methods are applied in specific cultural and geographic circumstances. The roads in rural Appalachia are long between towns. In central Appalachia, they ascend mountains and descend into valleys, while in urban northern Appalachia, they tend to be poorly maintained in the face of climate wear and budgetary priorities. In areas where population is sparse, the economic efficiency of clinics is suspect, and local hospitals, now almost exclusively maintained by large corporations run for profit, live under the steadily increasing threat of closure for underperformance.

Presented in Part Two are three scenarios: a comprehensive care clinic, telehealth networks, and grass-roots infrastructure building. Which offers the community more economic and educational development within itself? Which is cheaper to build and implement? If there is a difference between immediate results and playing a long game, does the intensity of Appalachia's short-term needs require sacrificing long-term development? There are no easy answers, but there are long-term possibilities, as these essays prove. The question is: which of these services, or what combination of them, is plausible to build, sustainable within the community, and best for the health of Appalachia's people?

Bob Franko discusses what is often called the Comprehensive Healthcare Delivery Model. In a national miasma of fragmented healthcare delivery, attempts to pull services together into a "no wrong door" model are more evolving than new. Health systems face many challenges as they look at ways to make sustainable billing systems, infrastructures, and administrative hierarchies to support such models, but they may also be cracking a problem that has dominated American public health for decades. Here, Franko discusses attempts to imbricate health care deliveries that have been seen as separate issues into better patient care delivery and smoother clinic operational methods. Is such blending the future of American health care in rural areas, where population sparseness dominates economic sustainability?

Steve North then examines what is arguably the fastest-growing model of healthcare delivery in rural areas: telehealth. North presents here case studies of several types of telemedical assistance delivered across different states, discussing their varying degrees of efficiency. He also gives a comprehensive look at the types of clinical needs best handled with telehealth, and what doctors in rural areas have observed about its best practice implementation. North concludes with ways in which telehealth's role is likely to increase over the next decade.

In what is perhaps a contrast to telehealth and parallel to comprehensive delivery, Marilyn Pace Maxwell and Tony Lawson tell the story of how one community's self-built integrated system is a win in several simultaneous directions. Mountain Empire Older Citizens, Inc., grew slowly and at a grass roots level from an eldercare facility into a multi-faceted community organization; it has since become an economic engine for growth in the region. This is what success stories look like when localities build for and within themselves the services they need for and within themselves: a true imbrication of culture, clinic and community that has stood the tests of time, funding crunches, and politics, because it was built on a solid, steady foundation of community need, muscle, and goodwill. The results not only deliver quality care to a needy community, but create an economic underpinning for other grassroots initiatives.

No examination of regional health would be complete without investigating the theories that have underpinned the overall public perception of that region. In Part Three, "Cultural Theory and Clinical Policy," contributors present three concepts that often drift unexamined into discussions of Appalachian health: patient responsibility, fatalism, and community based participation.

The line between blaming the victim and expecting personal responsibility from patients has been a blurry one for decades. Patient responsibility has appeared more subtly in the essays to this point, usually in the guise of individual behavior and personal choices. Wendy Welch and Esther Thatcher ask how unexamined constructs based on urban and majority populations add to the burden of stereotypes foisted onto rural areas, perhaps blocking effective health care delivery due to expectations. What happens if a person is limited to choosing between two bad options (e.g., refuse cancer treatment, or travel at significant cost and burden to one's family to receive it)? How much more difficult it is to plan and implement programs in a region where this holds true for some, but not all, citizens. Welch and Thatcher also posit whether corporations bear some burden of blame, perhaps even some financial responsibility, toward cleaning up messes to which they have contributed, while recognizing that such messes are caused in part by personal choices. They ask where personal responsibility ends and corporate begins — and who decides.

Fatalism has already reared its undefined head in prior essays in this volume. What does fatalism mean, and specifically how does it play out in the lives of young people in Appalachia? As Tauna Gulley explores fatalism and its counterpart, self-efficacy, she notes that family is a strong element of Appalachian life, often seen as one of the region's greatest assets. But perhaps in some ways the family dynamic discourages young people from developing healthy senses of self-esteem or self-efficiency. Perhaps the echoes of fatalism, so long a part of Appalachian stereotyping, actually reflected in the short-term views of the region's youth on their own health behaviors. Gulley explores this with fieldwork and academic research, concluding that family dynamics, while a force for the positive in many cases, must still be seen as a double-edged sword.

And finally, community-based participation, the active seeking of local wisdom and partnering with various stakeholders and influence wielders in geographic areas, has long been a one-size-fits-all catchphrase tossed about by funders, programmers, and policy makers alike. Does the phrase still have meaning, and in best and worst practice, what does community participation look like — and yield? Tom Plaut reflects on a lifetime of watching both best practice in community participation, and best laid plans gone awry. He ponders whether asking the right questions before beginning can lead to a straighter, more productive conclusion, and asserts that every voice has value. "A good measure of success in community research is what happens after a research project is completed," he suggests. Quiet voices sometimes get drowned out by assumptions — or even good intentions — but they are there, waiting to lend their inside perspective to the questions that affect their communities.

It was the aim of this volume of essays to provide multiple stories and internal observations that sometimes escape the mainstream, yet affect the way in which policies and programs roll out in Appalachia. The patchwork these various authors and their subject matter offer aim toward a holistic rather than a complete picture, avoiding simplifications and stereotypes while offering data, anecdotes, and analysis. If, as Tom Plaut observes in his concluding essay, the goal of health research is to improve the lives of those researched, then it is the fervent hope of those who contributed to this volume that their work does just that.

PART ONE:
HEALTH ISSUES

No Reason to Smile:
Dental Care in Rural Appalachia

SARAH RASKIN and A. CAROLE PRATT, DDS

It was already past closing time for the Missions of Mercy (MOM) free dental clinic on the fairgrounds in Wise County, Virginia, when the young man appeared at the dental triage tent. The volunteers had treated more than a thousand people with dental pain over two and a half days and were tired and sweaty, ready to take down the tents, load up the vans, and wind their way back down mountain roads to homes and offices and more familiar surroundings. They were ready to go back to where patients made appointments for regular dental checkups every six months, didn't sleep in their cars and trucks in the parking lot the night before, and might even be lucky enough to have a dental insurance policy through their jobs.

The young man was solemn, dressed in the dark olive uniform of the Virginia guardsmen and women who had been assigned to protect people and property and keep order at the large free clinic. He was slight in build and spoke politely when he asked if someone could take a look in his mouth. He thought maybe the dentists could do something for him before they all left. He had a toothache and it had hurt for as long as he could remember.

The volunteer dentist pulled on gloves, tied a mask over her face, grabbed a tiny mirror, and had him open his mouth. His teeth were easily as bad as any of the other patients the dental team had seen. He had several badly decayed and infected teeth with obvious swelling. Yes, the dentist could take a look. Yes, they would see if someone still had instruments that hadn't yet been packed so his dental pain could be treated.

As the young man walked away to have an x-ray taken to prepare for several extractions, another of his fellow guardsmen came to the dental tent. And another. And then another. These men and women all had regular jobs and had been awake through the night, standing guard at the tent city that is the Missions of Mercy dental clinic. They had toothaches and were not able to get dental insurance through their employment or afford treatment out of their pockets. Several guardsmen and women received dental treatment late that Sunday after most of the crowds of patients and volunteers had gone away.

There are many people at every Missions of Mercy clinic who are capable of taking one's breath away by the stories they tell: stories of lost jobs and poor health, of disappointments and missed opportunities, of just plain bad luck. But none of these situations seem any more unfair than knowing that men and women protecting the grounds while volunteers got a few hours of sleep, were standing guard while their teeth hurt.

Oral health and dental care in central Appalachia: the concept alone has become synonymous with problems and insufficiencies, disturbing images like "meth mouth" or derisive phrases like "toothless hillbillies." Headlines such as "At Appalachian Fairgrounds, Charity Tries to Fill Gaps in Health Care" (Sebert and Spolar 2009) call attention to the inadequacy of dental care in the region, while others like "Rot in Appalachia Deeper than Teeth" (*Lexington Herald Leader* 2009) and "In Kentucky's Teeth, Toll of Poverty and Neglect" (Urbina 2007) direct blame at its residents. Rare is the story that doesn't frame these issues, at least in part, in terms of culture. But what is a central Appalachian culture of oral health? Is it the charity clinic featured in the first passage, including patients who serve in our military and dentists who travel from elsewhere to treat them? Is it a local dental hygienist, who considers her job to be as much about health education as clinical services? At a time when the incidence of dental caries (cavities) has increased among ALL boys aged 2–8 in the United States and only 27.8 percent of low-income adults nationwide visits a dentist each year (Bailit et al., 2006) how can it be said that central Appalachia's statistics, some of which are indeed deeply concerning, are uniquely attributable to "culture"? This discussion is motivated by these and other questions. Insights are drawn from work in one central Appalachian sub-region, southwest Virginia, and from stories told by people who live there.

These stories are offered cautiously, because sharing more about central Appalachians' poor oral care risks being misunderstood as perpetuating some of the worst stereotypes circulated about the region and its residents. Some of these misconceptions include the idea that no one there has good oral health or adequate access to dental care and that the current situation is acceptable or unchangeable, all patently false notions. These stories can happen anywhere in the United States — and do. It is not only the alarming frequency with which they occur in central Appalachia that is of great concern, but also the clichéd ways they are told by a variety of people — jour-nalists, politicians, even neighbors who have better oral health and access to care — within and beyond the region.

Perhaps what distinguishes the people whose stories follow from those who have better oral health is their lack of access to resources both central and ancillary to getting care: paid leave time from work to be able to seek care and recover from procedures; working vehicles to travel to providers; a strong sense of self and belief in the idea that they can, will, and should be able to obtain a mouth that is both healthy and beautiful; and, of course, insurance coverage and money at hand to pay for all these things. It cannot be overstated that the single strongest predictor of oral health and access to dental care everywhere is socioeconomic status. So in an area such as southwest Virginia, characterized by higher-than-average rates of unem-ployment, low-wage or contingent work, and disability retirement, it fol-lows that oral health and access to dental care are both poor.

Yet we repeat the provocative claim that, in describing oral health and dental care in southwest Virginia, we are describing oral health and dental care in the United States. This microcosm, while certainly unique in terms of history and context, is not an anomaly, yet still is handled as such. And the region's plight is blamed, perhaps disproportionately, on individual behavior, including patient behavior such as home hygiene, and dental provider behavior, most notably where to locate a dental prac-tice. With this focus on individuals, systemic failures often go inadequately attributed, such as the ways in which oral health and dental care have been treated as separate from overall health and health care, or the woefully insufficient way that dental insurance is conceived, to the point that even people who have coverage oftentimes can't afford the high co-pays associ-ated with procedures. Most importantly, while the story of oral health and dental care in central Appalachia is particular and specific, it is neither the region's residents' fault nor their fate. To ground this claim in empirical evidence, the data in the following figure forms the framework that under-lies our premise.

What do these facts tell us about the situation of oral health and dental care in central Appalachia? On the one hand, they demonstrate that statistically the situation is worse than elsewhere. On the other hand, they offer little by way of explanatory power or description of the experiences of those suffering. In some ways they actually mask the problem more. For example, although up to 60 percent of far southwest Virginia's adults saw a dentist in the last year, they are more likely to have seen a dentist for an extraction or dentures than for routine examinations or cleanings. This information tells us that far southwest Virginia adults may be able to seek

Figure 1: Key Indicators in Oral Health and Dental Care			
	Far SWVA	*VA*	*US*
Adults who have had at least one permanent tooth extracted for decay or disease	58.7%	39.7%	43.9%
Adults who are "fully edentulous" (missing all teeth)	35%	unknown	10.5%
Adults who currently smoke	24.9–31.5%	18.5%	19.3%
Adults who have private dental insurance coverage	48.6%	69.6%	53.9%
Adult dental visitation in the past year for any reason	52.7–60.1%	70.7–76.4%	69.8–71.3%
Adults who report receiving regular dental cleanings	50%	70–75%	68.5%
Children in 3rd grade who have unresolved dental caries (cavities)	29.2–46.9%	15.4%	19.4%
Children who have dental insurance	88.6–87.5%	84.8%	77.2%
Children whose last dental visit was more than 3 years ago	9–10.6%	6.2%	2.8%
Children who were unable to get dental care or had an unmet need in the last year	7.1–11.6%	10.9%	2.8%
Private practice dentist/population	25/100,000	62/100,000	54.3/100,000
Percent of dentists whose patients primarily use private insurance	49%	70%	63.6%
Percent of dentists who accept Medicaid insurance	16.3%	4.3%	20%
Percent of patients who travel over 10 miles to dentist	45%	27%	21%
Sources listed in References; all figures pre–CHIP mandate			

treatments when they are needed, but still lack good access to preventive care.

Similarly, although up to 89 percent of far southwest Virginia's children have dental insurance, that statistic does not differentiate between private insurance and public insurance, despite our knowledge that type of insurance is predictive of access to care. (This is due to one's ability to find a dentist who takes that insurance.) Further complicating the interpretation of these statistics is our own experience and research. For example, far more than 11 percent of parents who participated in research by one of this essay's authors (Raskin) reported that their child had an unmet dental need. The figure of 25 dentists per 100,000 population is based on dentists who maintain a license with the state dental board and have a regional mailing address, although research (by Raskin) demonstrated that many of these dentists were in full or partial retirement. In order to offer a more nuanced perspective on these and other topics, we return to the stories of people affected by issues of oral health and access to dental care in the region. To get started, let us revisit the site of the first story.

One Kind of Clinic: The Charity Clinic

Anyone who wants to study problems surrounding oral health or access to dental care in central Appalachia can get a quick education by simply attending a free dental clinic, most of which are organized as Virginia Dental Association Missions of Mercy projects, or MOMs. The people who come for care and the problems they bring with them mirror the dental health crisis throughout the nation. A few patients are from distant states and even other countries, and the mere fact that they travel so far to stand in line for dental treatment at a fairground in the Appalachian Mountains defines the nature of the access problem.

But most live nearby in communities named Richlands, Elk Garden, Big Stone Gap, and Rosedale, pleasant-sounding places where many folks have run up against hard times. Layoffs and labor transitions have occurred as coal mines and manufacturers eliminated jobs. The more desirable manufacturing sector has largely been replaced by lower paying retail and service jobs, many without health care benefits or dental insurance.

It is not just the patients who have suffered. Populations in these towns have declined as many of the most educated and higher skilled residents moved away in search of better work. The people who remained lost the benefits of having them in their communities as individuals and population numbers, and the people who remained also lost purchasing power, along with the ability to hold professionals in the region to serve the dwindling population. Dentists lost patients, for lack of ability to pay and by population drop. This shift came about in the 1980s and '90s, when the debt load of new dental school graduates and costs of modern technologies rose.

Any dentist practicing in southwest Virginia or another economically depressed area now has to weigh economic factors against benevolent inclinations to provide some amount of free or reduced cost care. The ability to sustain a dental practice and dependably meet payroll weighs on the decision to locate in the region at all, rather than choosing a larger metropolitan area with more sustainable patient populations. Travel to a dentist in larger towns even an hour away can be difficult for many of the region's residents, either for lack of public transportation or a reliable family car. Yet that distance is what residents often have to travel for care. Much of southwest Virginia, like much of central Appalachia, is a federally designated Dental Health Professional Shortage Area, meaning that there are not enough dentists practicing in the region to provide adequate care for all of its residents.

It was within this context that Terry Dickinson, a dentist and Executive Director of the Virginia Dental Association, initiated the MOM projects. He recruited volunteer teams of dentists, dental hygienists, dental assistants, oral surgeons, and administrative staff to give a few days of service per year in temporary clinics set up in the region. The first MOM free dental clinic was held in 2000 at Lonesome Pine Airport in Wise County, in conjunction with another charity health care event, a Remote Area Medical (RAM) Expedition. Since then, the MOM project has served more than 16,000 people at its annual event at the Wise County fairground. MOM clinics are now held in all regions of Virginia and have been replicated in at least twenty other states across the country, sometimes in partnership with RAM's comprehensive medical clinics. They have served 47,000 people with donated care estimated at $29 million statewide. From the first project with 133 volunteers, the most recent clinic at Wise has grown to attract 378 volunteers from 14 states.

Treatment available at these mobile clinics has also expanded steadily. Early clinics offered basic dental services: examinations, cleanings, fillings, and extractions. By 2012, services had expanded to include digital x-rays, oral biopsies, root canal treatments, gross cleanings, fluoride varnishes, full and partial dentures, denture repairs and refittings, and more. All services are offered to the degree they can be made available given time and other resource constraints, including the great number of patients who seek to obtain them. Most of the dental patients come for what would be called emergency care in a private dental office — extractions or large restorations of teeth that have already become painful. Some patients come to obtain routine preventive dental care, such as a retired couple whose pensions did not provide enough for them to afford dental insurance. Their Medicare coverage did not extend to dental needs, but they knew the value of routine preventive care after years of attending MOM for extractions and other interventions.

Regardless of what they seek, all patients must wait in line to obtain a ticket, generally issued in order of arrival. Those who wait in long lines include healthy and young people, men and women with disabilities or in wheel chairs, people who carry their oxygen tanks, the working poor, and others whose presence is something of a surprise to volunteers — like the school nurse who works full time, is a single mother of three, and has no dental insurance. The clinic director reports as many as 70 percent of MOM dental patients are from a family where at least one person is employed full time but with no dental benefits. No one is questioned about insurance status or ability to pay, and as far as possible none are turned away. Although they are not asked, many of the clinic patients seem anxious to tell their stories and have someone understand why they come to the fairground for dental treatment. This seems especially true of the people whose needs are not able to be met by MOM. Such is the case of "Misty" (patient names are pseudonyms):

> As a first timer at the MOM Misty didn't realize that her only option would be to get her two bothersome teeth pulled, rather than getting the restorative care she'd hoped for. She'd had health insurance at her previous jobs — a factory that laid her off when she got pregnant and a customer service call center that closed — and Medicaid when she was pregnant with her daughter, but never dental coverage. Her daughter's father didn't contribute anything, and she couldn't afford to pay out of pocket for the crowns that she had hoped the MOM dentists could give her.
>
> Misty told me she lived with her parents so they could babysit while she attended community college to become a radiology tech. Then she started sobbing. "I'm about to enter the medical profession," Misty said, "How will patients take me seriously if I don't look like I take care of myself? Who wants a medical professional who looks like this?" She faced me directly for the first time in our conversation. She took her hand down from in front of her face where, I then realized, she'd been holding it to cover her mouth. Looking at her mouth, I wanted to make her feel better, to tell her that I'd seen far worse sets of teeth than hers. She seemed to still have all of her top teeth and the cracking and browning on them not as bad as others I'd met. Her breath didn't reek of old cigarettes or sugary carbohydrates or rotting — it was quite neutral, actually — and she had only one bottom tooth obviously missing. But that sort of platitude seemed unintentionally offensive. So I changed the topic [Field notes, SR, July 25, 2010 (edited for length)].

Dental extractions remain by far the most common treatment offered at MOM clinics. It would seem a better economic choice for a person to have the more costly root canal therapy that is also offered, but the specialists who do these procedures are sometimes unable to find MOMs patients to fill their chairs. People know that even though a root canal treatment will save their tooth, they would still need to have another high dollar procedure, a crown, after their root had healed — after the MOM had ended — and they cannot afford it. Having the tooth extracted seems an easier and certainly less expensive option for many.

Yet, as Misty's story illustrates, extraction of one or more teeth with little prospect of replacing them is a very hard choice for some patients to make. For them, having visibly missing teeth is too much to bear because of its implications for employability, social life, or just the way that people judge character. Unfortunately for people such as Misty, the alternative options are differently risky. Teeth and gum infections left unaddressed can have such consequences as increased risk for further pain, bone loss, complications with other diseases, and even death due to infection entering the blood stream. Conversely, the extraction of multiple teeth without restoration, which is often the only option available to MOM attendees with advanced decay and infection, can lead to jaw atrophy, misalignment of the teeth, and difficulty in chewing and speaking.

Among the lines of people waiting their turn in the dental chair, the majority are adults. Most dental and periodontal disease is preventable through proper home hygiene, good nutrition, and semi-annual dental visits for cleaning and examination, behaviors that ideally begin in childhood and are facilitated in a variety of contexts, both within the home and outside of it. This premise leads to the next clinical site and community of providers and patients: outreach to children at elementary schools.

The Clinic in the Community Setting: School-Based Preventive Dental Care

In 2000, the same year as the first MOM clinic, the Surgeon General released a comprehensive report on dental needs in the United States. National attention focused on what was named the "silent epidemic" of dental and oral disease. Dental decay, or cavities, was identified as the single most prevalent chronic disease of childhood, an alarming five times more common than asthma and seven times more common than hay fever. Yet one in four children from low-income families had not seen a dentist before they entered kindergarten. Over a decade after the Surgeon General's report, some improvements have been made but decay in children aged two to five has actually gone up. Less than half of Virginia's Medicaid eligible children see a dentist each year, even for an examination. The rest of the country's greatest asset — its children — fare no better. In 2009, only 44 percent of the more than 29 million Medicaid-enrolled children received any dental services. This is especially problematic given that, thanks to Medicaid, the Children's Health Insurance Program (CHIP) and health reform through the Affordable Care Act, America's children have a mechanism to cover basic dental services. However, simply being enrolled in one of the children's dental programs does not mean a child will get regular treatment or any treatment at all, especially in a region like southwest Virginia where there are simply not enough dentists to meet the population's needs, broadly or specific to a context in which burden of disease and coverage by public insurance are both high.

Sometimes children do not receive dental services because of parental or caregiver factors, a barrier to care that is not exclusive to southwest Virginia. However, one of the more urgent reasons that children have difficulty accessing dental services in southwest Virginia specifically is a lack of pediatric dentists. Special skill is required to treat small children, not all general dentists are comfortable treating them, and in southwest Virginia as in many other areas of the country, there are relatively few pediatric dentists. The Centers for Medicare & Medicaid Services have identified a number of reasons why so few dentists treat children covered by Medicaid and CHIP. Historically low reimbursement rates, complicated and time consuming billing procedures, patient failure to keep dental appointments, and transportation problems are cited, among others.

The inadequacy of dental care options for children in southwest Virginia in general, and children who are covered by public insurance in particular, has led to the development of some novel — if at times controversial — solutions. One is a pilot project allowing public health dental hygienists to deliver preventive care and patient education, services that can be delivered safely under the remote rather than on-site supervision of a dentist, to children in elementary schools.

> I accompanied the public health dental team to provide screenings, cleanings, fluoride rinses, sealants, education, free packets of toothbrushes, toothpaste, and floss, and referrals to eligible children at the elementary school. Because sealants were the emphasis of the program, I paid particularly close attention to the dental hygienist's decision whether to place sealants on each child's teeth. The story of the third patient who didn't receive sealants — Patient #4 — was uniquely captivating. Red-cheeked and crew-cutted, the boy wore a Spiderman shirt, no socks, and fatigue-print pants that were too short for him. The dental hygienist peered in his mouth for a long time, first just looking and then using

the dental mirror and probe gingerly. She tried to reassure him that she was "just counting his teeth" but his hands gripped the opposing forearms tightly. She asked him if it hurt. He nodded. Most of his teeth showed existing or imminent decay: sticky dark yellow plaque around his gum lines; dark vines of caries across the outer surfaces of seven teeth; black pits of decay in two molars, and puffy red gums around a third. The dental hygienist asked him when he had last seen a dentist. The boy responded meekly, "I don't remember." She probed, "Do you have a dentist?" "I don't think so," he responded. She asked him if he could remember the name of any dentist he'd ever seen. He couldn't. She later told me this was a sign that it had probably been way too long since he'd seen a dentist, if he ever had.

The dental hygienist told the boy she couldn't give him any services because his teeth needed "special treatment" (that is, to be cleaned and treated under anesthesia which she was not licensed to provide). She told him she was going to send home a note to his parents that he needed to see a dentist as soon possible, and that she would help him find one. At first, he didn't respond. Then he said that he didn't think his family would be able to take him to a dentist because his father was deceased and his mother permanently disabled and unable to drive. He explained that his uncle sometimes drove him places, but he couldn't depend on it. We four — the dental hygienist, the dental assistant, the school nurse, and I — looked among each other with a feeling of loss at what to do. The dental assistant took the boy aside to show him how to wipe his teeth with a paper towel and water after he ate breakfast and lunch at school while the dental hygienist and nurse conferred. A native of the community, the school nurse was familiar with the family and their tragic circumstances. She agreed with the boy's assessment that he was unlikely to be driven to a dentist, especially since the dentists who had agreed to see referrals were located at least a 45 minute drive away. The dental assistant loaded the boy's hands with as many toothbrushes and tubes of toothpaste as he could carry, figuring he'd wind up distributing them to equally needy family members if he couldn't use them himself. The school nurse agreed to keep a close eye on him and contact the dental hygienist if his teeth seemed worse, or if he seemed in immediate pain or danger of infection because of them. Together, they might be able to work out one visit to the dentist, even if it meant one of them driving him. One visit. For emergencies only. But what about the next time, or the time after that? Their guess was as good as anyone's [Field notes, SR, Nov 22, 2010 (edited for length)].

Dental outreach initiatives that emphasize prevention such as this one have been demonstrated to be safe and cost effective (Day 2011). The dental outreach team gives critical clinical services to some of the children most at risk for dental disease, but it also provides two other important services: teaching children good behavioral habits and socializing them in the experience of receiving dental care as a way to reduce fear. However, programs such as this are not without flaws that threaten their effectiveness. One of the biggest obstacles is the low response rate among parents, for reasons that are not yet well understood.

Another obstacle is the limitation of time. Outreach staff travel far distances to schools only to be limited in their ability to provide services by the duration of the school day and curricular and social mandates, such as a ban on calling children in for services during periods of lunch and statewide testing preparation. A third obstacle is the limitation of this outreach project to the public health sector, by law, when it could be scaled up to safety net and even private clinics. A fourth obstacle to success is the inadequacy of the referral network. As discussed, few local dentists are able and willing to see children who are insured by Medicaid; thus it becomes the time-consuming task of public health dental outreach staff to identify and negotiate with providers, urging them to see the children with the most urgent needs. Lastly, another obstacle is the nature of the professions themselves. As in many other fields, organized dentistry has been reluctant to support the broadening of tasks from dentists or dental auxiliaries working in dentists' offices to other settings in which mid-level providers may work semi-autonomously, despite evidence from a variety of settings worldwide demonstrating that a reallocation of specific minimally-invasive tasks — most, prophylactic — can be provided safely and to tremendous public health effect.

The Clinic of Last Resort: The Emergency Room

As limited as the options are for children needing dental care, those for adults are worse. Medicaid is the public health insurance program for those with limited incomes, funded jointly by state and federal governments and managed by the states. Dental coverage is mandated for children who receive Medicaid benefits, but not for adults. In recent years Medicaid dental benefits for adults have been reduced or eliminated by many states as a way to reduce expenses in tight budget times. Virginia's dental care for adult patients is meager, covering only medically necessary care like emergency extractions. Thus, for some, the option of last resort is the hospital emergency room.

Hundreds of thousands of Americans seek dental care in emergency rooms every year. Across the country 830,590 emergency room visits in 2009 were for preventable dental conditions, a number that has risen by an alarming 16 percent since 2006 (Pew 2012). This option is unsatisfactory for several reasons, not least the lack of long-term resolution to the dental complaint. The patient will probably leave with two prescriptions, one for antibiotics and another for pain medication, along with a referral to see a dentist. A referral to a dental clinic isn't even as valuable as the paper it is written on for someone who lacks the funds, time, transportation, or other resources to access a dentist.

A more likely scenario is that the patient will take the prescriptions, the tooth will get better after a few days, and if the person is lucky, she will be pain-free for some weeks. Sooner or later, without fail, the tooth will hurt again, and the cycle starts all over. This scenario may make that person more vulnerable to addiction to pain medicine or more likely to try risky self-treatment like prescription pain medicine borrowed from others, illicit drugs, or even extracting her own tooth. Southwest Virginia's reputation as a place where addiction to prescription medicine runs rampant has caused some emergency rooms to reject the appeals of someone suffering from dental pain outright, even when he or she is not seeking narcotic pain medicine. One dental patient, Mike, described the ways in which this problem breaks down trust and causes a withholding of services between providers and patients:

> You tell them you've got a toothache. Then they take one look at you and see that you're poor, and they think you're there to get pain pills. So they turn you out, tell you they can't help you. Tell you to go see your dentist on Monday. Man, I just lanced my own abscess and drained all sortsa nastiness out of it. If I wanted pain pills, I'd go ask my cousin. I'm here for antibiotics! But they see you up in the E.R. on a Saturday night trying to have them look in your mouth and they think one thing: He's a junkie [Mike, Interview with SR, November 10, 2010].

As Mike indicates, even this dental clinic of last resort is becoming less available over time, as hospitals close emergency rooms due to lack of funds, or decide to turn away dental patients as a blanket policy to avoid dealing with the issue of drug-seeking. Where will patients turn when their emergency system of care is as inaccessible as the traditional dental care system?

Provider Prospects

The future of dental care in southwest Virginia is literally in the hands of those who chose to practice in these communities. In this difficult practice environment, why do dentists choose to locate here, and why do young people from the area want to go away to dental school and return? Historically, fewer dentists choose practice sites in rural areas than in more urban locations. This is even more problematic for Virginia, which according to the American Dental Association ranked 34th for the number of dental students enrolled per 100,000 people even though it is the 12th most populous state. The following are a collection of thoughts from current and future dentists who are drawn to practice in this region at least in part because of the opportunities to help address the problem of limited access to dental care.

A senior student at the University of Virginia's College at Wise writes this in her application to dental school:

"How are you doing?" I asked a 20-year-old woman as I escorted her from the dental triage to the extractions tent at the Remote Area Medical (RAM) event in Wise, Virginia.

"My family drove eight hours, we camped out last night and I've been awake since 3:00 a.m. It's not that bad though," the woman replied. "I am just happy to be here."

The young woman did not even flinch when [the dentist] told her she would need a full mouth extraction due to her extensive caries. During the laborious procedure, [he] paused to reassure the patient. A tear rolled down her cheek and without hesitation I grabbed her hand. She said, "Honey, it's not the pain. I am so grateful and appreciate everything you all do." It was at this moment that I knew I wanted to be a dentist.

A dental student from southwest Virginia, now at Virginia Commonwealth University, tells how he is drawn back to his home:

I have no doubt that growing up in southwestern Virginia has impacted the way that I view dentistry. If nothing else, my experiences have helped me to realize the impact dentistry can make in the lives of others. Even as I write, I can't help but remember the countless smiles and expressions of gratitude of the patients I've been fortunate enough to interact with during my experiences both in private practice and during MOM Projects. It's because of their appreciation that, to me, dentistry will never feel like "work."

In addition, my experiences have given me perspective as a dental student. As I learn about the prevalence of oral disease in southwestern Virginia, I cannot help but rely on my own experiences to understand the bigger picture. In some instances, dentists are avoided because of the notion that dentistry must be painful. In other instances, patients don't understand the importance of oral hygiene or consider dental work an unnecessary expense. Unfortunately, few even make the assumption that they will inevitably lose all their teeth and need dentures, and make the decision to neglect their oral health. For these reasons, and many more, I'm passionate about oral health education and about the health disparities of southwestern Virginia.

Interests in health policy and a passion for the health disparities and the oral health of residents of southwestern Virginia will continue to shape my career and where I decide to practice. With that said, it is, and has always been, my intention to return to southwestern Virginia to practice dentistry. Although I can't account for what the future may hold, I can't imagine not giving back to the area that I consider to have already given me so much.

A relatively new dentist practicing in southwest Virginia had reservations about coming to a rural area but now feels lucky to call the mountains home. She and her husband came to live in his childhood hometown and this is how she came to love it:

> Before we married, we decided that upon finishing dental school I would be the one to make the move to join him in his part of the state. Interestingly enough, my final year of school I was assigned a clinical rotation exactly where my husband and I planned on settling down. It was on this rotation that I fell in love with a place I would soon be proud to call home and discover just how much I enjoyed serving those around me through my career in dentistry.
>
> Perhaps one of the best things about settling down in this area has been the incredible career and service opportunities I've been given. At first I was concerned that I may not have all the same opportunities to learn and grow that I might have been afforded in a larger city; however, having the ability to work side by side every day with one of the best prosthodontists in the area, I truly feel as though I've been getting my own version of a one-on-one residency. Because of him, I've been able to work with everything from implants to crown and bridge to one of the latest denture techniques in the country. Over the last year he's inspired me to become an active member of our local dental society and participate in numerous mission projects in the underserved areas around us. These service projects have turned out to be one of the most fulfilling aspects of my career here. This particular region of the state has many areas where access to care is an major issue, so to be able to help those in need, many who live not far from my own backyard, has been such a blessing.

This dental specialist has practiced in southwest Virginia, his childhood home, since 2001. In addition to holding leadership roles in dental organizations and mentoring recent dental school graduates, he plays a prominent role in the MOM free dental clinics by directing the team providing denture services. The son of a coal miner and a factory worker, he tells why practice in southwest Virginia was the only choice for him:

> I was the first college graduate on both sides of our family and the first to break the coal mining legacy. I understand the people of southwest Virginia and I have family living in poverty. The folks I know are people dedicated to their families and their jobs. I do not remember my father missing a day of work in 28 years. He was the smartest man I have ever met throughout my life. He taught me how to think and was a great example of how to reflect the light that God has given you. The proudest day of my life was in February 2001 when he and my mother were able to see me open my own prosthodontic practice in Bristol, Virginia.
>
> I grew up in a small town called Honaker, Virginia. It is surrounded by coal mining communities. My father-in-law is the coal mine manager for the same company where my father was employed. He resides in Grundy, Virginia and that location is the site for the October Mission of Mercy Project. It is one of three projects I volunteer for with the Virginia Dental Association. The other two projects occur in Wise, Virginia in July and Roanoke, Virginia in March. I am co-director of the Denture Team for the VDA MOM projects. This team is comprised of volunteer dentists and lab technicians from within the state. These projects treat the uninsured and underinsured from our area and many

other states. The number of people at these projects seeking care seems to grow with every passing year. The common theme that exists is that of unemployment and no money to get the much needed medical and dental care. Many of my family and patients in coal mining and related businesses have lost their jobs due to what they call "The War on Coal." This in combination with the lack of education on how to prevent dental and medical problems has created a growing access to care issue in our communities. The number of people without any teeth and the ability to chew continues to rise with each passing MOM project. Currently, our waiting list for people needing dentures has risen to over 400 with new names being added every day. I feel very blessed to have the opportunity to restore a person's ability to smile and chew. In the last two years, our denture team has delivered over 500 complete arches of teeth to those less fortunate. However, the edentulous rate continues to rise at an even greater number with each passing project. Our communities need to be on fluoridated water sources and our country needs to return the manufacturing jobs to these communities.

Finally, there is the story of how dental need in southwest Virginia has reached a California oral surgeon turned entrepreneur, who developed a new, one-step denture method that he introduced at one of the Virginia MOM clinics. The new streamlined approach is an economical alternative to the traditional, more costly and more time consuming dentures, and is being welcomed by free clinics and many dental schools across the country. Here is how the technique was brought to central Appalachia:

> I was in Oral Surgery private practice for 25 years, took out thousands of teeth, and I saw the devastation: emotionally, physically, and psychologically of taking out all of one's teeth ... I went to (a southwest Virginia dentist's) office and we did twelve dentures on six patients.... Three months later I'm at my first MOM clinic.

He goes on to say that the most gratifying part of the process is

> seeing the absolute joy in the face of the patients who get their dentures, and knowing we're fulfilling a real need. Those needs are there, not only at MOM projects, but also in our private offices ... giving back is always something I wanted to do.

These people are part of the solution to the problem of oral health and dental care in southwest Virginia. But the largest barrier to dental care is financial, and that will not change no matter how many dentists locate nearby. For new dental school graduates, the decision to practice dentistry in central Appalachia or in any other underserved area in the country is a complex one. These communities are ones with high rates of unemployment and low rates of private dental insurance. According to the American Dental Association, dentists have an average of $177,144 in educational debt alone upon graduation. Ability to pay off debt is no small consideration in where they decide to practice, and may discourage new dentists from practicing in underserved areas. The American Dental Association has identified a steady trend towards group rather than solo practice. The preference for this type of practice eliminates some rural opportunities, where solo practice predominates. Other proposed solutions must be considered as well.

Proposed Solutions

Evidence suggests that dentists are more likely to choose to practice in rural or underserved areas if they themselves are from those communities, or if they are given the opportunity to serve them early in their training. Fully half of southwest Virginia's dentists surveyed recently said they chose a practice location because it was close to where they grew up. Even though only 37 percent of them graduated from Virginia's single dental school, 60 percent were graduates of a local or regional high school (Rephann et al., 2011).

In an effort to meet the demand for dentists in underserved areas of the state, Virginia's only dental school has increased its class size by twenty students over the last decade, and sets aside places for students identified as being from areas of dental need. In addition, consistent with national trends to co-locate dental care with the medical safety net, the dental school has established a practicum opportunity for dental students with a Federally Qualified Health Center in the region. Although it is too soon to know if the results of these strategies will be borne out in the short or long term, they demonstrate creative approaches to cultivating a more sustainable variety of dental care options.

Another area that is undergoing reform is the relationship between medicine and dentistry. Led by the Virginia Oral Health Coalition, a new medical/dental collaboration initiative draws on the national Smiles for Life curriculum to serve both oral and systemic health needs by utilizing dynamic practice models, such as pediatricians' application of topical fluoride and dental staff screening for diabetes risk. Other Coalition successes with implications for patients in southwest Virginia include helping to develop a statewide oral health plan and advocating for restoring funding of the state's dental safety net programs, including MOM projects.

Advocates continue to work to increase dental reimbursement rates for Medicaid, and streamline administrative practices for CHIP and Medicaid in order to incentivize dentists to participate more in these programs. In addition, they work to maintain the dental safety net by providing services for children and adults in public health, free clinic, and community health center settings, as well as maintain the delivery of the most impactful public dental health service of all — fluoridated water — to their entire community. Finally, they continue to work on strategies to implement and evaluate activities that have an impact on health behavior, promote interventions to reduce tooth decay and associated risk behaviors, and evaluate and improve methods of monitoring oral diseases and conditions.

The most transformational project to address oral health needs in central Appalachia was announced on a clear autumn morning in 2012 on the slope of a mountain in Tazewell County, Virginia. Community leaders and health care professionals gathered at The Bluestone Business and Technology Center to hear plans for a new dental school, a public-private partnership among Bluefield College, Tazewell County, and the Tazewell County Industrial Development Authority.

The views that day were the kinds that make one stop and notice: misty blue mountains, the suggestion of cinnamon on the tips of some dogwood leaves, lazy grasshoppers making the most of vanishing summer, nothing at all to suggest the coming dental school campus. The announcement itself was opened and closed by fervent prayers, and vision in the Old Testament sense was mentioned more than once. Those who for years dreamed of such a school in this remote area of the state have a goal of meeting the oral health needs of the area while creating hundreds of direct and indirect new jobs for the professors and support staff that such a program will require.

"Dentists and professional dental care are limited in central Appalachia, but this new dental school will address that problem and begin to fill our understaffed clinics with the personnel needed to provide rural residents with sufficient oral care," said Dr. David Olive, president of Bluefield College. Plans are for third and fourth year students to learn and work in rural clinics. Student recruitment will be heavy in rural Southside and southwest Virginia, with expectations that some of the graduates will return to these communities or ones like them to establish practice.

Supporters are enthusiastic while naysayers shake their heads. Their list of obstacles is a long one: not enough patients for all categories of treatment students must learn, budget worries, difficulties recruiting faculty, challenges with the community-based learning model. But which is harder to imagine: a dental school at the foot of a mountain, or thousands of people coming from all parts of the United States to get teeth fixed at the MOM clinic at a fairground where last week there was a livestock show?

Conclusion

Dr. Risa Lavizzo-Mourey, president and CEO of the Robert Wood Johnson Foundation, the nation's largest health philanthropy, said in a recent essay that a child's life expectancy is predicted more by ZIP code than genetic code. The same can be argued about a person's dental health. The single highest predictor of whether a person will seek dental care in any given year is whether they are covered by dental insurance. In southwest Virginia's ZIP codes, where unemployment has reached the highest level in decades and the area's rate of job loss has been more severe than elsewhere in the country, the outlook for dental care access looks bleak.

Although lack of health care access is a high price to pay, many southwest Virginians say they wouldn't live anywhere else. They enjoy a relatively low cost of living, beautiful outdoor recreation areas, an unhurried pace of life, a strong and creative cultural tradition, vibrant communities of faith and family, and a reasonably short drive to a number of urban areas. Like other rural Americans, residents have a more difficult time accessing the full range of health services, including dentistry. In a country that pairs health insurance benefits with employment, and with job loss in the region more acute than the rest of the country, the decision to live and work here often comes with the realization that there may be no dental or medical benefits available.

On the backs of the volunteers at MOM dental clinics, shirts bear this quote from Buddhist nun Pema Chodron, "We didn't set out to save the world; we set out to wonder how other people are doing and to reflect on how our actions affect other people's hearts." This simple quote is a rallying call for those who believe that free dental care at a MOM clinic, no matter how selfless the volunteers are or how many patients are being treated, cannot solve the problem of growing dental needs in central Appalachia — or across the country. If the words on these shirts are taken literally, then the volunteers must surely have learned that some "other people" are not doing nearly as well as they would hope. Depending on the generosity of a caravan of volunteers who sometimes travel hundreds of miles to practice their professions in an airplane hangar or at a county fairground is not a sustainable answer to the so-called silent epidemic of dental disease.

"I realized my mission was to focus on bringing help to those who struggle every day to put food on the table, to pay rent, to put gas in the gas tank," said Dr. Terry Dickinson, the dentist and Virginia Dental Association Executive Director who founded the MOM programs. "MOM programs have provided care to those who need it the most, but the lack of access to oral health care continues to be a problem in this country.

Dentists can do what they can to help, but ultimately the federal, local and state governments and society at large must stop shortchanging oral health and find the political will to get better dental care to the millions of Americans who need it" (Crozier 2009). No longer the silent epidemic of oral and dental disease the Surgeon General warned the nation about in 2000, the problem is literally crying out to be heard.

Part of the research that contributed to this essay was funded by the National Science Foundation Doctoral Dissertation Research Improvement Award #0961762 and the Agency for Healthcare Research and Quality Dissertation Research Award #R36 HS19117.

References

American Dental Association. N.d. http://www.ada.org/.

American Dental Education Association. N.d. http://www.adea.org/.

Bailit, H., Beazoglou, T., Demby, N., McFarland, J., Robinson, P., and Weaver, R. 2006. "Dental Safety Net: Current Capacity and Potential for Expansion." *Journal of the American Dental Association* 137, no. 6 (June).

Crozier, Stacie. 2009. "Missions of Mercy Is His Life's Mission." *ADA Newsletter*, December 22. http://www.ada.org/news/434.aspx (accessed 21 July 2013).

Day, Karen. 2011. Virginia Department of Health Dental Hygiene Pilot. Paper presented at the Virginia Oral Health Coalition Summit October 21 in Richmond, VA. http://www.vaoralhealth.org/wp-content/uploads/2010/10/Karen-Day.pdf (accessed 1 September 2012).

Du Molin, Jim. 2011. Dental Patients and How Far They Travel. http://thewealthydentist.com/surveyresults/059-dental-patient-travel-distance.htm (accessed 25 June 2012).

Health Resources and Services Administration. N.d. Oral Health Workforce homepage. http://www.hrsa.gov/publichealth/clinical/oralhealth/workforce.html (accessed 14 January 2012).

The Kaiser Family Foundation, statehealthfacts.org. Data Source: Centers for Disease Control and Prevention, Behavioral Risk Factor Surveillance System Survey Data (BRFSS) 2010. Unpublished data (accessed 12 October 2012).

Lexington Herald-Leader. 2009. Op-Ed: "Rot in Appalachia Deeper than Teeth." 23 March: A7.

National Survey of Children's Health. 2003. Child and Adolescent Health Measurement Initiative, Data Resource Center on Child and Adolescent Health website. http://childhealthdata.org/browse/survey/results?q=1205 (accessed 25 October 2013).

National Survey of Children's Health. 2007. Child and Adolescent Health Measurement Initiative, Data Resource Center on Child and Adolescent Health website. http://childhealthdata.org/browse/survey/results?q=1205 (accessed 25 October 2013).

The Pew Charitable Trusts, State and Consumer Initiatives. 2012. A Costly Dental Destination: Hospital Care Means States Pay Dearly. http://www.pewstates.org/research/reports/a-costly-dental-destination-85899379755 (accessed 5 August 2012).

Rephann, Terance J., Shobe, William M., and Wanchek, Tanya. 2011. Oral Health and the Dental Care Workforce in Southwest Virginia, a Report of the Weldon Cooper Center for Public Service Center for Economic and Policy Studies, University of Virginia. http://www.coopercenter.org/econ/publications/oral-health-and-dental-care-workforce-southwest-virginia (accessed 30 October 2012).

Schaller-Ayers, J., and Ayers, J.W. 2007. Health Care Access in Southwest Virginia: A Technical Report. Wise, VA.

Sebert, Lagan, and Spolar, Christine. 2009. "At Appalachian Fairgrounds, Charity Tries to Fill Gaps in Health Care." *Common Dreams*, August 8, http://www.commondreams.org/headline/2009/08/08-2 (accessed 28 September 2012).

Urbina, Ian. 2007. "In Kentucky's Teeth, Toll of Poverty and Neglect." *New York Times*, December 24, http://www.nytimes.com/2007/12/24/us/24kentucky.html? pagewanted= all&_r=0 (accessed 4 August 2012).

Vargas, Clemencia M., Crall, James J., and Schneider, Donald A. 1998. "Sociodemographic Distribution of Pediatric Dental Caries: NHANES III," 1988–1994. *Journal of the American Dental Association* 129, 9: 1229–1238, cited in Rephann, Shobe, and Wanchek 2011.

Virginia Department of Health. N.d. Tobacco Indicators by Health District. http://www. vdh.state.va.us/ofhs/prevention/tucp/data.htm (accessed 25 October 2012).

Wendling, Wayne. 2009. The Private Practice of Dentistry, a Presentation to Institute of Medicine Workshop: Sufficiency of the U.S. Oral Health Workforce in the Coming Decade. http://www.iom.edu/~/media/Files/Activitypercent20Files/Workforce/oralhealth workforce/2009-Feb-09/1percent20-percent20Wendling.pdf (accessed 12 November 2011).

Cancer in Appalachia

Morgan Fields, Gretchen E. Ely, and Mark Dignan

Cancer is a group of diseases characterized by disruption in the regulation of cells in the body. The disruption alters the way that cells divide and are replaced (cell death, in other words) and results in development of a population of tumor cells with the ability to invade other tissues (Ruddon 2007).

The Appalachian population has a higher burden of cancer than the rest of the United States. (In this essay, Appalachia refers to what is sometimes called central, mountain or Coalfields Appalachia: primarily West Virginia, Virginia, Tennessee and Kentucky, with perhaps parts of rural North Carolina.) Table 1 shows the incidence rates (new cases diagnosed in a given year) and mortality rates (deaths from cancer per year) for the most common cancer types in the Appalachian and non–Appalachian population for the period 2002–2006. As Table 1 shows, the rate at which new

Table 1. Incidence and Mortality Rates, Selected Cancers, Appalachia compared to Non-Appalachia, 2002–2006 (Appalachia Community Cancer Network 2010)				
	Appalachia		Non-Appalachia	
	Incidence	Mortality	Incidence	Mortality
All Cancer Sites	2900.5	1242	2398	975.7
Female Breast	702.5	153.6	617.4	129.4
Cervical	53.6	16.3	40.1	12.2
Colon & Rectum	336.1	121	262.4	98
Lung & Bronchus	502.3	393.5	371	288
Prostate	859.1	152.9	779	136.4
Rates are per 100,000 population				

cancer cases are diagnosed and the rate of death from cancer are both substantially higher in the Appalachian population.

Figures 1 and 2 illustrate the difference in cancer burden between Appalachia and the rest of the U.S.

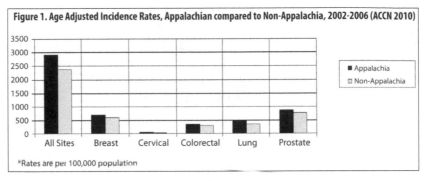

Figure 1. Age Adjusted Incidence Rates, Appalachian compared to Non-Appalachia, 2002-2006 (ACCN 2010)

*Rates are per 100,000 population

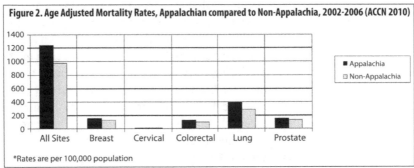

Figure 2. Age Adjusted Mortality Rates, Appalachian compared to Non-Appalachia, 2002-2006 (ACCN 2010)

*Rates are per 100,000 population

Factors Influencing Cancer Rates in Appalachia

Many factors contribute to the higher rates of cancer incidence and mortality in Appalachia. These factors can be organized into four basic categories: individuals and their behaviors, cultural factors, access to health services, and environmental factors.

Individuals and Their Behaviors

Individual factors include genetic heritage and behaviors. The elevated rates of cancer in Appalachia are undoubtedly related to genetics. Science and medicine are just beginning to understand how to study genetic factors, so in the future there will be much greater awareness of how genetics influence disease and how to use genetic information to combat cancer. For the present, a family history of cancer is an important indicator of increased risk. It is an accepted truism that individuals with blood relatives who have had cancer are at higher risk than the general population. Further, the greater the presence of cancer in one's family history, the greater the risk.

In previous generations, the Appalachian population was relatively isolated. Isolation over time results in the concentration of the genetic characteristics of a population. Such concentration can influence risk of various diseases, including some cancers. Genetic factors provide important clues about the elevated cancer rates in Appalachia, even though the Appalachian population today is not nearly as isolated as it was in previous generations.

A number of behaviors are associated with cancer risk, but none is so well documented as tobacco use — mostly smoking. Tobacco use is a major risk factor for cancer, as well as for other chronic diseases (Siegel 2012; Weiss 1997). Studies within the Appalachian region indicate that up to 50 percent of primary care patients report some sort of tobacco use (Behringer 2006). Smoking has been identified as a behavior that is closely related to other cancer risk factors, but the only factor that makes smoking even worse is low rates of adherence to cancer screening recommendations (Amonkar 2002). Smoking accounts for 30 percent of all cancer deaths and 87 percent of lung cancer deaths in the U.S. (Appalachia Community Cancer Network 2010).

West Virginia, the only state that lies entirely within Appalachia, has an adult smoking prevalence rate of 26.8 percent (Centers for Disease Control and Prevention 2010). The national rate of adult smoking prevalence is almost 10 percent less at just 17.3 percent (Centers for Disease Control and Prevention 2010). Also associated with tobacco use is living below poverty level and lack of education, both of which are noted socioeconomic disparities in the Appalachian region (Kruger 2012).

Other behaviors, including poor diet and lack of exercise, are also linked to increased cancer risk in Appalachia. Excessive weight is the second leading cause of preventable death in the U.S. population; this excessive weight is even more pronounced in the Appalachian region (National Institute of Diabetes and Digestive and Kidney Diseases of the National Institutes of Health 2005; Kentucky Department for Public Health 2005). Some studies show that overweight and obesity may account for up to 20 percent of cancer (van Kruijsdijk 2009).

Measures of overweight and obesity are defined in terms of Body Mass Index (BMI). The BMI is determined by using a calculation of an individual's height and weight. An individual who is overweight has a BMI between 25 and 29.9 and an individual who is obese has a BMI of 30 or greater (Centers for Disease Control and Prevention 2012a). History of obesity has also been associated with lack of compliance with cancer prevention seeking (Amonkar 2002).

In West Virginia, only 67.1 percent of individuals reported participation in physical activities in the last month, compared to 76.1 percent of the U.S. overall population (Centers for Disease Control and Prevention 2010). Similarly, 35 percent of West Virginia residents (per BMI) are overweight and 32.9 percent are obese (Centers for Disease Control and Prevention 2010). The U.S. rates of overweight are 36.2 percent and the rate of obesity is 27.5 percent (Centers for Disease Control and Prevention 2010).

Cultural Factors

Attitudes toward health and prevention that are considered unique to the Appalachian population may contribute to the way cancer plays out in the region. Religious faith and fatalistic attitudes could contribute to health service seeking behaviors in the area (Royse 2011). Religion probably plays a role in whether individuals choose to be screened or treated for cancer in the first place. Also, in order to understand a diagnosis like cancer, people turn to frameworks they are comfortable with such as religious beliefs (Behringer 2011). In Appalachia, more than 50 percent of the population self-identifies with a faith community (Behringer 2011). These religious Appalachian residents may hold fatalistic beliefs about a cancer diagnosis; in other words, they may turn to their spirituality to guide the outcome of their disease.

However, religion is not a simple issue in this situation. A reliance on faith may lead some patients to not investigate other opinions, or to seek or even avoid alternate therapies (Behringer 2011). Others may use their spiritual beliefs to help get them through the diagnosis and treatment in a more supportive manner (Behringer 2011). Fatalism can also be viewed as a reflection of the experience with cancer in this population, where most patients have historically succumbed to their disease. Fatalism is also likely to be a reflection of the despair stemming from a diagnosis when associated with poverty, the high cost of cancer care, and a lack of insurance (Royse 2011).

Patients with a cancer diagnosis have noted the importance of religion as a coping mechanism. Unfortunately, the majority of physicians, as well as others on the medical care team, have not received any education on religion (Behringer 2011). This puts researchers at a disadvantage in interpreting how religion affects patients, and it puts providers at a disadvantage; when religion plays a great role in their patients' care, it may put distance between them and their patients (Behringer 2011).

Research suggests that, given the low educational attainment of many residents of Appalachia, a lack of awareness of cancer, of cancer screening procedures, and of publicly supported breast and cervical cancer public health efforts may influence cancer rates. Information further suggests that Appalachian residents most often gain cancer related information from friends, neighbors and relatives, rather than from health providers (Behringer 2006), a cultural factor that may sometimes frustrate doctors, but which they would do well to not overlook when speaking with patients.

In addition to the cultural reliance on familiar voices over non-familiar ones, and on family wisdom over incoming professionals, independence is an important cultural characteristic of the Appalachian population, and one that may influence experience with cancer. The independent nature may be manifested in terms of decisions to forego specialty care if it cannot be obtained locally.

Access to Health Care

Limited access to health care services is a challenge faced by many rural communities. Appalachian counties typically have lower population density when compared to the rest of their state (Behringer 2006). The area is also characterized by geographically remote communities that lack access to health providers (Behringer 2006) and are generally considered medically underserved (Lengerich 2004). This isolation may also affect residents' ability to seek preventive cancer testing and other health services (Behringer 2006). There are also generally fewer health care providers in these communities, and thus fewer health care facilities, especially specialty services (i.e., MRI, OB/GYNs, Oncologists, etc.) (Punglia 2006; Chan 2006; Arcury 2005; Jones 2008). Having fewer providers and facilities means that residents of these areas must choose from those available or travel long distances for their health care needs (Maheswaran 2006).

The need to travel long distances in order to receive cancer screenings has been linked with later stages of cancer diagnoses (Huang 2009). Additionally, insurance companies may limit coverage to specific providers, thus forcing these individuals to have to travel to get their cancer health care needs covered (Huang 2009). Such travel is often difficult for these residents due to their low levels of income and the lack of accessible transportation (Arcury 2005; Maheswaran 2006; Celaya 2006). Additionally, individuals living in Appalachia are less likely to have health insurance in the first place, and thus cannot afford to pay for cancer screenings or cancer treatments if diagnosed (Royse 2011). This may be one of the reasons they often choose not be screened (Royse 2011).

Another reason these individuals are not screened may be because of low literacy and low health literacy, both of which are relatively prominent in the region due to lower levels of formal education (U.S. Department for Health and Human Services 2000; Institute of Medicine 2004; Berkman 2011; Berkman 2010).

Environmental Factors

There are many environmental factors associated with cancer risk that can be found in the Appalachian region. Some examples of these environmental causes are exposure to chemicals, radiation, and high levels of pollutants (Appalachia Community Cancer Network 2010). Appalachian communities have often been exploited for their natural resources. Residents identify concerns that toxic waste; runoff from farms, mines, and factories; unclean water; and occupational hazards may impact the cancer risk and health seeking behaviors in this region (Behringer 2006).

Results from a recent study suggest that individuals who live not only in Appalachia but specifically in areas where coal mining takes place are at an even greater risk for health disparities, including higher rates of cancer mortality (Hendryx 2012). This is especially true in coal mining areas that utilize "mountain top mining" or "mountain top removal" strategies (Hendryx 2012). The study also indicates that individuals living in these mountain top mining areas of Appalachia were twice as likely to have cancer than those living in an area of Appalachia with no mining (Hendryx 2012). One explanation for this phenomenon is increased exposure to environmental carcinogens such as Arsenic, Chromium and Cadmium. That translates into 1.2 million residents of Appalachia's mountaintop mining areas being at double the risk for developing cancer, in comparison to the United States population overall (Hendryx 2012).

Strategies for Reducing the Cancer Burden in Appalachia

Reducing the cancer burden in Appalachia requires focusing on the natural history of cancer and using strategies to prevent cancer from developing, detecting cancer early in its development, using state-of-the-art treatments in cases where cancer has developed, addressing issues of cancer survivors including rehabilitation, and providing palliative care. Efforts to prevent cancer from developing are termed "primary prevention." Detection of cancer early in its development is "secondary prevention," and providing treatment to prevent death from cancer is "tertiary prevention."

Primary Prevention

A growing arsenal of strategies to prevent cancer exists. These strategies start with interventions to impact behaviors and reduce exposure to known cancer-causing substances (carcinogens). They also include application of procedures to detect and remove precancerous cells, and — most recently — the application of a vaccine.

Tobacco

Perhaps the best example of a strategy to reduce exposure to carcinogens is prevention of tobacco use and the promotion of tobacco cessation. In recent years there have been many smoking cessation campaigns targeting Appalachian residents. The effort to promote smoking cessation has come at the same time that the region has seen a dramatic reduction in the number of tobacco-producing farms. The reduction in farming tobacco has resulted in less economic dependence on income from tobacco (Kruger 2012). This decrease in dependence makes it more acceptable for health advocates and residents to be outspoken against tobacco use (Kruger 2012).

In recent decades, there has been an increase in Internet and cable use in the Appalachian region (Kruger 2012). This facilitates greater access to health information, including facts about the detriments of tobacco use and facts about the benefits of tobacco cessation. The opinions of family and friends on tobacco in Appalachia are an indicator of how residents perceive tobacco use and cessation (Kruger 2012). If an individual's family and friends support someone who is trying to quit smoking or chewing, the individual is more likely to be able to succeed in quitting (Kruger 2012).

Evidence also suggests that the support of an individual's health care provider is a key component in successful smoking cessation (Kruger 2012). Bans on smoking in public places have been growing in popularity and evidence supports that the bans effectively reduce smoking, not to mention exposure to second-hand smoke (Kruger 2012). In fact, Appalachian states such as Tennessee have enacted state-wide smoking bans designed to protect the health of residents; these bans suggest that many people now acknowledge that smoking is an issue affecting the public health. Therefore, this may be an option for Appalachian communities wishing to reduce tobacco use. However, support of the community, as mentioned above with friends and family, is key to ensuring the success of such a ban (Kruger 2012).

Obesity

A growing body of evidence suggests that obesity increases cancer risk (van Kruijsdijk 2009; National Institute of Diabetes and Digestive and

Kidney Diseases 2005; Kentucky Department for Public Health 2005; Amonkar 2002; Centers for Disease Control and Prevention 2010). Accordingly, there have been several different types of interventions developed to reduce obesity in the United States. In 2009, the CDC released "Recommended Community Strategies and Measurements to Prevent Obesity in the United States" (Khan 2009). Many of these strategies are applicable to Appalachian communities. Increasing access to affordable and healthy food and drink in communities is one method (Khan 2009). One way of implementing this has been shown in Kentucky, where an individual may use their Special Supplemental Nutrition Program for Women, Infants, and Children (WIC) benefits at farmers markets and other local health food stores, in order to increase intake of fresh produce and locally grown food (Kentucky: Cabinet for Health and Family Services).

Another strategy mentioned by the CDC is to use schools as a place to encourage healthy eating and physical activity (Khan 2009). The school should provide lunches and snacks that are healthy, and should include a physical education requirement (Khan 2009). The school should also promote and encourage extracurricular physical activity (Khan 2009).

Similarly, communities themselves should facilitate physical activity for residents (Khan 2009). In an ideal world with funding to provide safe pathways, this can be done by promoting walking and bicycling as a mode of transportation, as well as for recreational use (Khan 2009). Also, communities with publicly accessible recreational facilities should promote use of these facilities to residents by expanding hours and/or programs offered (Khan 2009); this might not apply to many Appalachian rural settings, but where possible it would assist. Lastly, communities should be advertising changes made to the community to promote physical activity and nutrition, and allowing residents to become involved in the efforts to create a healthier community (Khan 2009).

Human Papilloma Vaccination (HPV)

Research indicates that the human papillomavirus (HPV) facilitates the development of cervical cancer (Bosch 2003; Schiffman 1995). In fact, a high risk HPV infection that facilitates a cervical abnormality must occur in order for the abnormality to progress into cervical cancer (Centers for Disease Control and Prevention 2012b). While the Pap test (as it is known) remains the standard procedure for identifying the presence of precancerous and cancerous cells on the cervix, the development of an HPV vaccine that prevents contraction of several strains of HPV identified with cervical cancer is an important step in the prevention of the disease (Centers for Disease Control and Prevention 2012b). In particular, vulnerable populations of women living in medically underserved areas, such as Appalachia, where the Pap test is not regularly and consistently used, could benefit most from widespread uptake of the vaccine (Hopenhayn 2007; Bach 2010).

The burden of cervical cancer mortality differs greatly between higher and lower income groups of women (Bach 2010). Women who have the greatest access to Pap tests and the subsequent treatments are typically in higher income groups, and have better access to the vaccine, while lower income women who have the most compromised access to Pap testing and treatments are also the least likely to receive the vaccine during the recommended age of initiation (Akers 2007). Recent research indicates that having a higher cervical cancer mortality rate predicts a lower vaccination rate, as does residing in a state with a lower median income (Centers for Disease Control and Prevention 2009). Such information indicates that the most medically compromised populations are the least likely to receive the vaccine.

Invasive cervical cancer rates have been found to be highest in the Appalachian states of Kentucky and West Virginia (Hopenhayn 2008). The rate of cervical cancer in Kentucky is 10.3 per 100,000 people in the fifty-four county Appalachian region of Kentucky, compared to a rate of 8.61 in all other Kentucky counties (Kentucky Cancer Registry 2012). Appalachian young women have great potential to benefit from widespread diffusion and uptake of the HPV vaccine because of the elevated incidence and mortality rates of cervical cancer in their region (Hall 2000; Hopenhayn 2008; Katz 2009). While the vaccine is available through the federally funded Vaccines for Children program (VFC) recent studies indicate that the vaccine is not being used in populations most in need of it, namely, those who are the poorest and most medically underserved (Bach 2010). Thus, there is a profound need for increased cervical cancer prevention and screening efforts in Appalachian counties in Kentucky.

While cervical cancer incidence and mortality rates have declined in general over the last several decades in the United States, rates in populations of Appalachian women have actually increased (Hopenhayn 2005, 2008; Lengerich 2005). The FDA approved the vaccine in 2006 to prevent four strains of HPV, which causes 70 percent of cervical cancer (Munoz 2006; Walboomers 1999). With this availability comes the opportunity to vaccinate a population against the contraction of a type of cancer for the first time in history. Such an opportunity is most important for vulnerable populations, as high risk HPV infection — the kind that often leads to the development of cervical cancer — is most prevalent in poor women in the United States, especially in the Appalachian region (Kahn 2007).

Evidence suggests that parental attitudes and life experiences influence attitudes towards acceptability of HPV vaccination for their daughters (Dempsey 2006). In light of the uniqueness of the life and parenting experiences in central Appalachia, efforts to increase cancer screening and preventive health behaviors must be tailored to the region (Ely 2010). As one example, the region can be characterized as socioeconomically disadvantaged, and high-risk HPV infections are associated with lower socioeconomic status (Kahn 2007) so prevention efforts should be tailored to the needs of families who experience economic vulnerability. Also, in light of the dearth of health facilities, alternative locations for health screenings and interventions must be considered. Cancer screening and prevention in Appalachia needs to be promoted as available in local communities through local providers, which makes cancer related health behaviors seem achievable, rather than perceived as only available at expensive, distant health centers (Behringer 2006). Neither of these touches on the issue of religion, discussed earlier with regard to cancer treatment generally. Pap tests and cervical vaccinations can be a hotbed of discussion points for discerning cultural scholars.

Secondary Prevention — Early Detection Through Screening

Secondary prevention, more commonly referred to as "screening," currently includes procedures to detect changes associated with the development of breast, cervical, colorectal and prostate cancers. Specific screening tests are available for each of the following types of cancer.

Breast Cancer Screening

Screening for breast cancer is designed to detect breast tumors early in their development. Finding breast tumors when they are small and have not spread to other parts of the body provides the best chance for successful treatment. Breast cancer screening includes clinical breast exam and mammography (Appalachia Community Cancer Network 2010).

Mammography is the best method to use to find and diagnose breast cancer early (Appalachia Community Cancer Network 2010). Breast cancer affects both women and men, but is much more common in women. In Appalachia, the rate of women receiving a mammogram in the past two years is 3.2 percent lower than the U.S. rate, at just 68.6 percent (Hall 2002). Similarly, the rate of women who have received a clinical breast exam in the past 2 years is 75 percent, 2.5 percent lower than the U.S. rate (Hall 2002). Women who have lower income, less educational attainment, worse health status, or who are unemployed, uninsured, and/or smoke have been found to be those most likely to not have routine breast cancer screening (Hall 2002).

Cervical Cancer Screening

As mentioned previously, screening for cervical cancer is done through a Pap test (Appalachia Community Cancer Network 2010). Pap tests involve collection of samples of cells from the cervix during a pelvic exam. Examining the cells allows identification of changes that indicate the impending development of cancer or the presence of cancer. Women in Appalachia have not only higher rates of cervical cancer but also lower rates of Pap testing (Hatcher 2011). The rate of invasive cervical cancer for Appalachian women is about 40 percent higher than the U.S. rate (Schoenberg 2009). Individuals at highest risk for cervical cancer are those who have never had Pap tests or who do not get screened routinely (Hatcher 2011). An intervention has been developed and implemented among Appalachian women to combat exactly this. The community-based participatory research intervention, titled "Faith Moves Mountains," has been effective in educating Appalachian women about cervical cancer screening and assisting in keeping them up-to-date with their screening (Hatcher 2011; Schoenberg 2009).

Colorectal Cancer Screening

Recommended screening for colorectal cancer occurs through testing for blood in stool or through visual inspection of the inside of the colon with sigmoidoscopy and/or colonoscopy (Appalachia Community Cancer Network 2010). In terms of cost, early and routine screenings not only save money but also reduce mortality. It has been found that, "Colorectal screenings that cost on average $125 can identify cancer before symptoms appear, after which the cost is approximately $100,000 with a survival rate of only 8 percent" (Shell 2004). In Appalachian Kentucky, only 36 percent of the population is current with their colorectal cancer screenings, in comparison to 53 percent of the U.S. (Bardach 2012). Research also showed that among Appalachian Kentucky residents, in statistical analysis and after controlling for many factors, knowledge about screening recommendations (i.e., frequency of screenings) remained significant as to whether an individual was compliant with their screenings (Bardach 2012). This suggests that by increasing knowledge of screening recommendations, colorectal cancer screening rates will also increase.

In general, individuals living in the Appalachian region are less likely to receive cancer screening tests of any type (Appalachia Community Cancer Network 2010). The reasons include limited access to preventive health

care that promotes screening, limited awareness of screening, and — similar
to most populations — a lack of recommendations from health care providers to obtain screening (Appalachia Community Cancer Network 2010).

Other reasons stem from the socioeconomic characteristics of the
population and the Appalachian culture. A high proportion of the population is low income and many do not have either health insurance or
funds that can be used for prevention. Scarce resources must be conserved
for providing food and shelter and for health-related emergencies. Also,
the Appalachian culture values independence and self-reliance; many distrust "outsiders and their ways"— including health care providers from
outside the region. While these cultural values reinforce the resilience of
the population, they may also work against cancer prevention and early
detection.

Finally, in experiencing high cancer rates, the Appalachian culture,
like many cultures, has become accustomed to cancer patients succumbing
to their disease. As one individual from Appalachian Kentucky stated, "I
don't think that Eastern Kentucky [Appalachia] is educated about the survival rate for those that catch it early. Cancer itself is perceived as a death
sentence. Why would you go looking for it? That's the last thing you want
is to go looking for it if you don't think there's anything you can do about
it anyways" (Schoenberg 2012).

Efforts to Increase All Types of Cancer Screening in Appalachia

Strategies that have been, are, or may be employed to increase cancer
screening in Appalachia include:

1) local individuals from community-based organizations leading efforts to
improve cancer screening awareness and to change attitudes regarding cancer
prevention; 2) use of specific communication strategies (such as newspapers,
churches, and community leaders) to help people get accurate cancer screening
information, reinforcing the importance of talking to health care providers about
cancer screening, and decreasing the amount of cancer-related information that
is misunderstood; 3) best practices to improve provider-patient communication
about cancer screening; and 4) system-level activities which are put into place,
such as chart reminder systems to help health care professionals remind people
to get cancer screening and follow-up, and changes to health care systems to
provide needed cancer screening services to the population by establishing local
or mobile cancer screening units to serve more rural regions of Appalachia
[Appalachia Community Cancer Network 2010].

Other recommendations to improve screening rates are the use of storytelling from a community member who has been diagnosed with cancer,

increasing knowledge of family history of cancer, increasing publicity for the organizations and resources available in and to the community, and establishing a "one stop shop" for screenings, allowing patients to receive multiple screenings in one day at the same location (Schoenberg 2012). In speaking about having known someone with cancer or someone who has received a screening exam, one woman talked about her reason behind getting a Pap test: "It's not as scary as everyone thinks it is. I went with my friend when she was having one, and it lasted maybe 5 minutes. Then I decided to have one after she talked to me, and having the nurse there too helped. She was patient and let me feel the equipment and told me what she was doing and went through every step" (Schoenberg 2012).

Lastly, one individual spoke about a novel idea for screening: "Wouldn't it be great if employers would just say that you have a day during the year to go and get screened and it would not count against your pay or your banked time? Just to give people the time to go and get screened…. The employers would benefit just as much as the person…. Also, if you took a friend or co-worker to get screened then you would get a day off just for helping out" (Schoenberg 2012).

Treatment for Cancer in Appalachia

In many parts of the United States, those who are diagnosed with cancer have several options for treatment. In rural Appalachia, the range of options is more limited. Initial surgery for the most common cancers is often available in many Appalachian community hospitals, but follow-up chemotherapy and radiation are less likely to be available. Patients must often travel hundreds of miles to obtain chemotherapy and even farther for radiation therapy.

When individuals from the Appalachian region are diagnosed with cancer, making decisions about treatment is very difficult. It is characteristic of Appalachian residents to consult with their family members who have a large influence on their ultimate decision (Coyne 2006). They often want to stay close to their family members, so even if better treatment is available outside the community, when their family cannot travel with them, they will often decide to obtain cancer treatment closer to home and to their family (Coyne 2006; Kannapel 1999; Wilson 1997). Related to treatment are Appalachian residents' decisions on whether or not to participate in clinical trials. Overall, residents of rural areas are less likely to participate in clinical trials (Baquet 2006). It is believed that this is also in relation to the patient's family and friends' influences (Schoenberg 2003).

Living with Cancer

After receiving a cancer diagnosis, Appalachian residents may be unsurprised and fairly accepting of the information (Hutson 2007). This acceptance may be due to the "storytelling" that occurs in the region (Hutson 2007). This storytelling includes stories of cancer, and as one individual stated, "[community members] expect to get [cancer]. They all do. It's almost like it's inevitable" (Hutson 2007). One researcher added, "When stories passed from one generation to the next, fear and anxiety appeared to be transferred, thereby passing along cancer screening beliefs and behaviors" (Hutson 2007).

Appalachian patients may also be distanced from the health care system because of their lack of trust in healthcare and physicians (Hutson 2007). They often report feeling stereotyped in medical settings and that they are often overlooked in the system (Hutson 2007). This feeling may be due to patients' fatalistic beliefs, lack of insurance, or the lack of rapport between patient and provider (Hutson 2007). Because of these feelings, patients not only feel distanced, but also have low expectations of the health care system (Hutson 2007). This only exacerbates the likelihood that Appalachian residents will continue their avoidance of both cancer screenings and treatment (Hutson 2007).

The Future

What is to be done to reduce the cancer burden in Appalachia? It is often said that if the problem is in the community, then the solution is in the community. With this concept in mind, current and future efforts to curb the cancer problem must begin with active participation by the community. The local public brings to this process the knowledge of community assets, barriers to prevention and early detection through screening, and barriers to gaining access to cancer treatment. The health care provider community brings knowledge of the challenges of developing and maintaining high quality health care for a population with scarce financial resources. Bringing these communities together is essential to create long-lasting, trusting relationships between those with resources and the usually guarded Appalachian community (Schoenberg 2012).

References

Akers, A.Y., Newmann, S.J., and Smith, J.S. 2007. "Factors Underlying Disparities in Cervical Cancer Incidence, Screening, and Treatment in the United States." *Current Problems in Cancer* no. 31: 157–181.

Amonkar, M.M., and Madhavan, S. 2002. "Compliance Rates and Predictors of Cancer Screening Recommendations among Appalachian Women." *Journal of Health Care for the Poor and Underserved* no. 13 (4): 443–460.

Appalachia Community Cancer Network. 2010. "Addressing the Cancer Burden in Appalachian Communities."

Arcury, T.A., Preisser, J.S., Gesler, W.M., and Powers, J.M. 2005. "Access to Transportation and Health Care Utilization in a Rural Region." *Journal of Rural Health* no. 21: 31–38.

Bach, P. 2010. "Gardisil: From Bench, to Bedside, to Blunder." *The Lancet* no. 365: 963–964.

Baquet, C.R., Commiskey, P., Daniel-Mullins, C., and Mishra, S.I. 2006. "Recruitment and Participation in Clinical Trials: Socio-demographic, Rural/Urban, and Health Care Access Predictors." *Cancer Detection and Prevention* no. 30 (1): 24–33.

Bardach, S.H., Schoenberg, N.E., Fleming, S.T., and Hatcher, J. 2012. "Relationship between Colorectal Cancer Screening Adherence and Knowledge among Vulnerable Rural Residents of Appalachian Kentucky." *Cancer Nursing* no. 35 (4): 288–294.

Behringer, B., and Friedell, G. 2006. "Appalachia: Where Place Matters in Health." *Preventing Chronic Disease* no. 3 (4): A113.

Behringer, B., and Krishnan, K. 2011. "Understanding the Role of Religion in Cancer Care in Appalachia." *Southern Medical Journal* no. 104 (4): 295–296.

Berkman, N., Ohene-Frempong, J., McCormack, L., and Davis, T.C. 2010. "Health Literacy: What is it?" *Journal of Health Communication* no. 15 (S2).

Berkman, N.D., Sheridan, S.L., Donahue, K.E., Halpern, D.J., Viera, A., Crotty, K., Holland, A., Brasure, M., Lohr, K.N., Harden, E., Tant, E., Wallace, I., and Viswanathan, M. 2011. "Health Literacy Interventions and Outcomes: An Updated Systematic Review." In *Evidence Report/Technology Assessment*. Rockville, MD.: Prepared by RTI International — University of North Carolina Evidence-based Practice Center under contract No. 290-2007-10056-I.

Bosch, F.X., and de Sanjose, S. 2003. "Chapter 1: Human Papillomavirus and Cervical Cancer-Burden and Assessment of Xausality." *Journal of the National Cancer Institute Monographs* no. 31 (1): 3–13.

Celaya, M.O., Rees, J.R., Gibson, J.J., Riddle, B.L., and Greenberg, E.R. 2006. "Travel Distance and Season of Diagnosis Affect Treatment Choices for Women with Early-stage Breast Cancer in a Predominantly Rural Population (United States)." *Cancer Causes and Control* no. 17: 851–856.

Centers for Disease Control and Prevention. 2009. "National, State, and Local Area Vaccination Coverage among Adolescents Aged 13–17 Years — United States." *Morbidity and Mortality Weekly Report* no. 58: 997–1001.

_____. 2010. Behavioral Risk Factor Surveillance System.

_____. 2012a. Division of Nutrition, Physical Activity, and Obesity. 2012, http://www.cdc.gov/obesity/index.html.

_____. 2012b. HPV Information for Clinicians. May, http://www.cdc.gov/STD/hpv/STD Fact-HPV-vaccine-hcp.htm.

Chan, L., Hart, L.G., and Goodman. D.C. 2006. "Geographic Access to Health Care for Rural Medicare Beneficiaries." *Journal of Rural Health* no. 22: 140–146.

Coyne, C.A., Demian-Popescu, C., and Friend, D. 2006. "Social and Cultural Factors Influencing Health in Southern West Virginia: a Qualitative Study." *Preventing Chronic Disease* no. 3 (4): A124.

Dempsey, A.F., Zimet, G.D., Davis, R.L., and Koutsky, L. 2006. "Factors that are Associated with Parental Acceptance of Human Papillomavirus Vaccines: A Randomized Intervention Study of Written Information about HPV." *Pediatrics* no. 117 (5): 1486–1493.

Ely, G.E., Flaherty, C., Cook-Craig, P., Dignan, M., White, C.R., Good, S., and Deskins, S. 2010. "A Case Study of Health Risk Behaviors in a Sample of Residents in Rural Appalachia." *Contemporary Rural Social Work* no. 10: 32–44.

Hall, H.H., Rogers, J.D., Weir, H.K., Miller, D.A., and Uhler, R.J. 2000. "Breast and Cervical Carcinoma Mortality among Women in the Appalachian Region of the U.S.: 1976–1996." *Cancer* no. 89: 1593–1602.

Hall, H.I., Uhler, R.J. Coughlin, S.S., and Miller, D.S. 2002. "Breast and Cervical Cancer Screening among Appalachian Women." *Cancer Epidemiology Biomarkers & Prevention* no. 11: 137–142.

Hatcher, J., Studts, C.R., Dignan, M., Turner, L.M., and Schoenberg, N.E. 2011. "Predictors of Cervical Cancer Screening for Rarely or Never Screened Rural Appalachian Women." *Journal of Health Care for the Poor and Underserved* no. 22 (1): 176–193.

Hendryx, M., Wolfe, L., Luo, J., and Webb, B. 2012. "Self-reported Cancer Rates in Two Rural Areas of West Virginia with and without Mountaintop Coal Mining." *Journal of Community Health* no. 37: 320–327.

Hopenhayn, C., Bush, H., Christian, A., and Sheldon, B.J. 2005. "Comparative Analysis of Invasive Cervical Cancer Incidence Rates in Three Appalachian States." *Preventive Medicine* no. 41: 859–864.

Hopenhayn, C., Christian, A., Christian, W.J., and Schoenberg, N.E. 2007. "Human Papillomavirus Vaccine: Knowledge and Attitudes in Two Appalachian Kentucky Counties." *Cancer Causes and Control* no. 18 (6): 627–634.

Hopenhayn, C., King, J.B., Christian, A., Huang, B., and Christian, W.J. 2008. "Variability of Cervical Cancer Rates across 5 Appalachian States: 1998–2003." *Cancer Causes and Control* no. 113: 2974–2980.

Huang, B., Dignan, M., Han, D., and Johnson, O. 2009. "Does Distance Matter? Distance to Mammography Facilities and Stage at Diagnosis of Breast Cancer in Kentucky." *Journal of Rural Health* no. 25 (4): 366–371.

Hutson, S.P., Dorgan, K.A., Phillips, A.N., and Behringer, B. 2007. "The Mountains Hold Things In: The Use of Community Research Review Work Groups to Address Cancer Disparities in Appalachia." *Oncology Nursing Forum* no. 34 (6): 1133–1139.

Jones, A.P., Haynes, R., Sauerzapf, V., Crawford, S.M., Zhao, H., and Forman, D. 2008. "Travel Time to Hospital and Treatment for Breast, Colon, Rectum, Lung, Ovary and Prostate Cancer." *European Journal of Cancer* no. 44: 992–999.

Kahn, J.A., Lan, D., and Kahn, R.S. 2007. "Sociodemographic Factors Associated with High-risk Human Papillomavirus Infection." *Obstetrics & Gynecology* no. 110: 87–95.

Kannapel, P.J., and DeYoung, A.J. 1999. "The Rural School Problem in 1999: A Review and Critique of the Literature." *Journal of Research in Rural Education* no. 15: 67–79.

Katz, M.L., Reiter, P.L., Kluhsman, B.C., Kennedy, S., Dwyer, S., Schoenberg, N., Johnson, A., Ely, G.E., Roberto, K., Lengerich, E.J., Brown, P., Paskett, E.D., and Dignan, M. 2009. "Human Papillomavirus (HPV) Vaccine Availability, Recommendations, Course and Policies among Health Departments in Seven Appalachian States." *Vaccine* no. 27: 3195–3200.

Kentucky: Cabinet for Health and Family Services. 2012. *WIC Farmers Market Nutrition Program*. Available from http://chfs.ky.gov/dph/mch/ns/FMNP.htm.

Kentucky Cancer Registry. 2012. *Age Adjusted Cancer Incidence Rates in Kentucky: Cervix Uteri, 2003–2007 by Appalachian Region*. Cited May 1, 2012. Available from http://cancer-rates.info/ky/index.php.

Kentucky Department for Public Health. 2005. The Kentucky Obesity Epidemic.

Khan, L.K., Sobush, K., Keener, D., Goodman, K., Lowry, A., Kakietek, J., and Zaro, S. 2009. "Recommended Community Strategies and Measurements to Prevent Obesity in the United States." *MMWR* no. 58 (RR07): 1–26.

Kruger, T.M., Howell, B.M., Haney, A., Davis, R.E., Fields, N., and Schoenberg, N.E. 2012. "Perceptions of Smoking Cessation Programs in Rural Appalachia." *American Journal of Health Behavior* no. 36 (3): 373–384.

Lengerich, E.J., Tucker, T.C., Powell, R.K., Colsher, P., Lehman, E., and Ward, A.J. 2005. "Cancer Incidence in Kentucky, Pennsylvania and West Virginia: Disparities in Appalachia." *Journal of Rural Health* no. 21: 39–47.

Lengerich, E.J., Wyatt, S.W., Rubio, A., Beaulieu, J.E., Coyne, C.A., Fleisher, L., Ward,

A.J., and Brown, P.K. 2004. "The Appalachia Cancer Network: Cancer Control Research among a Rural, Medically Underserved Population." *The Journal of Rural Health* no. 20 (2): 181–187.

Maheswaran, R., Pearson, T., Jordan, H., and Black, D. 2006. "Socioeconomic Deprivation, Travel Distance, Location of Service, and Uptake of Breast Cancer Screening in North Derbyshire, UK." *Journal of Epidemiology and Community Health* no. 60: 208–212.

Munoz, N., Castellsague, X., de Gonzalez, A.B., and Gissman, L. 2006. "HPV and the Etiology of Human Cancer." *Vaccine* no. 24: 1–10.

National Institute of Diabetes and Digestive and Kidney Diseases. 2005. National Diabetes Statistics Fact Sheet: General Information and National Estimates on Diabetes in the United States. Bethesda, MD: U.S. Department of Health and Human Services.

Nielsen-Bohlman, L., Panzer, A.M., and Kindig, D.A. (eds). Health Literacy: A Prescription to End Confusion. Institute of Medicine Committee on Health Literacy. Washington, DC: National Academies Press: 2004.

Punglia, R.S., Weeks, J.C., Neville, B.A., and Earle, C.C. 2006. "Effect of Distance to Radiation Treatment Facility on Use of Radiation Therapy after Mastectomy in Elderly Women." *International Journal of Radiation Oncology, Biology, Physics* no. 66: 56–63.

Royse, D., and Dignan, M. 2011. "Fatalism and Cancer Screening in Appalachian Kentucky." *Family Community Health* no. 34 (2): 126–133.

Ruddon, R.W. 2007. *Cancer Biology.* 4th ed. New York: Oxford University Press.

Schiffman, M.H., and Brinton, L.A. 1995. "The Epidemiology of Cervical Carcinogenesis." *Cancer* no. 76: 1888–1901.

Schoenberg, N.E., Amey, C.H., Stoller, E.P., and Muldoon, S.B. 2003. "Lay Referral Patterns Involved in Cardiac Treatment Decision Making among Middle-aged and Older Adults." *Gerontologist* no. 43 (4): 493–502.

Schoenberg, N.E., Hatcher, J., Dignan, M.B., Shelton, B., Wright, S., and Dollarhide, K.F. 2009. "Faith Moves Mountains: An Appalachian Cervical Cancer Prevention Program." *American Journal of Health Behavior* no. 33 (6): 627–638.

Schoenberg, N.E., Howell, B.M., and Fields, N. 2012. "Community Strategies to Address Cancer Disparities in Appalachian Kentucky." *Family and Community Health* no. 35 (1): 31–43.

Shell, R., Tudiver, F. 2004. "Barriers to Cancer Screening by Rural Appalachian Primary Care Providers." *Journal of Rural Health* no. 20 (4): 368–373.

Siegel, R., Naishadham, D., and Jemal, A. 2012. "Cancer Statistics, 2012." *CA: A Cancer Journal for Clinicians* no. 62: 10–29. doi: 10.3322/caac.20138.

U.S. Department for Health and Human Services. 2000. With Understanding and Improving Health and Objectives for Improving Health. Healthy People 2010. Washington, D.C.: U.S. Government Printing.

van Kruijsdijk, R.C., van der Wall, E., and Visseren, F.L. 2009. "Obesity and Cancer: The Role of Dysfunctional Adipose Tissue." *Cancer Epidemiology Biomarkers & Prevention* no. 18 (10): 2569–2578.

Walboomers, J.M., Jacobs, M.V., Manos, M.M., Bosch, F.X., Kummer, J.A., and Shah, K.V. 1999. "Human Papillomavirus is a Necessary Cause of Invasive Cancer Worldwide." *Journal of Pathology* no. 189: 12–19.

Weiss, W. 1997. "Cigarette Smoking and Lung Cancer Trends. A Light at the End of the Tunnel?" *Chest* no. 111: 1414–1416.

Wilson, S.M., Henry, C.S., and Peterson, G.W. 1997. "Life Satisfaction among Low-income Rural Youth from Appalachia." *Journal of Adolescence* no. 20 (4): 443–459.

The Growing Problem
of Diabetes in Appalachia

CARL J. GREEVER, MD, RACHEL WARD
and CHRISTIAN L. WILLIAMS

While known for its beautiful mountains and its relative isolation from the rest of the country, Appalachia is also characterized by poverty and high rates of chronic disease, including diabetes. A number of factors influence the general poor health of this region. Unhealthy dietary behaviors, such as high intakes of sugar-sweetened beverages, a shift away from physically active lifestyles, and limited access to health care all play roles in the diabetes burden experienced by residents of Appalachia. In this chapter, we will review diabetes, its determinants and effects, and how this disease has disproportionately impacted Appalachia compared to the rest of the United States. We will also discuss the region's cultural strengths, particularly the strong role of the family unit in decision-making, which could be harnessed to improve the diabetes outcomes of its communities.

Definition

Diabetes is a disease of impaired regulation of blood levels of glucose. The human body requires glucose in order to function and it must maintain the concentration in the blood within certain limits. If the level drops too low, the brain does not function well; if the level continues to drop, coma and death can result. When blood glucose levels start to rise, the body secretes more insulin, which causes some of the glucose to be converted into glycogen and then stored. If the glycogen storage system becomes full, the glucose is converted into fat. As blood glucose levels drop, the body converts stored glycogen back into glucose in order to bring levels back up. If glycogen stores are depleted, the body can convert muscle protein to glucose.

In diabetes, the process keeping the blood glucose from getting too high is impaired. This may be due to a lack of insulin secretion and/or an overload from too much ingestion of carbohydrates. This impairment can also stem from a lack of proper response by end organs. This is called insulin resistance.

There are actually two different types of diabetes; they are distinct yet similar diseases. Type I diabetes is when the pancreas fails to secrete enough insulin. This usually begins early in life and is called juvenile diabetes. Type II diabetes usually begins later in life, often as an adult and is called adult onset diabetes. Type II diabetes is much more sensitive to environmental factors and is far more common than Type I. Type II diabetes will be the focus of this discussion.

The consequences of the elevated levels of blood glucose and insulin are usually gradual, and related to the degree of elevation and the length of time the elevated levels persist. Diabetes can affect the circulatory system by accelerating the process of artery hardening (called atherosclerosis). This can lead to heart attacks, strokes, and blockages of peripheral arteries, which may result in amputation. Also, elevated levels of glucose and insulin can increase the risk of hypertension or high blood pressure, which has a negative effect on blood flow.

Diabetes can cause damage to the kidneys and lead to the need for dialysis and transplants. Diabetes can lead to damage to the eye, resulting in blindness. Diabetes may also affect the peripheral nervous system and immune system, resulting in increased falls, issues with mobility, and a reduced resistance to infections respectively. These isssues are often irreversible and life threatening as well as very expensive for both the individual and society.

Causes

The alarming, nationwide increases in diabetes have been linked to changes in lifestyle, especially eating patterns and — to perhaps a lesser extent — exercise patterns. Many studies have shown that people eating high fiber and low calorie foods have a relatively low incidence of diabetes, as well as other diseases common in Western dietary regions. As individuals increase their caloric intake, usually through foods that are low in fiber and nutrients, the incidence of diabetes increases. These increases have reached the point that the impact on health care expenditures has received the attention of political leadership and government budget makers.

The causes of diabetes can be divided into genetic and environmental. While there is much research being conducted by geneticists, at the present time, we are unable to use genetics as a tool for treatment or prevention. Therefore, we must concentrate on environmental factors. These are primarily physical activity and diet composition. It is well established that a sedentary lifestyle predisposes one to diabetes. Energy metabolism during physical activity is slightly different from basal metabolism and this is less stressful on the glucose regulation mechanism. Probably more important from our perspective is diet, as evidence exists that dietary changes, if started early enough, can reverse and/or prevent diabetes.

Public understanding of nutrition varies widely. Books on foods, nutrition, cookbooks and diet advice abound; there are books on high carb diets, low carb diets, high fat diets, low fat diets, vegetarian diets, juice diets, gluten-free diets, vegan diets, paleo diets, calorie restricted diets, diets bearing the names of prestigious medical clinics and health newsletters, and diets bearing the names of un-bashful authors thriving on publicity. Most, if not all, of these books claim to be based on evidence — or at least strong opinions about facts that justify their position. Is it any wonder that nutritionist Paavo Airola chose the title *Are You Confused?* for his book? This plethora of seemingly contradictory information has made it very difficult to understand the true roots of the problem.

From a medical perspective, diet has been an important component of diabetes treatment for many decades. There has been some ongoing controversy about the ideal proportion of carbohydrates, proteins and fats in the diet. As our understanding of nutrition has developed, it has become apparent that all carbohydrates are not nutritionally equivalent. Just as there are important differences in proteins and various fats, there are subtle differences in the way the body metabolizes different carbohydrates, even if they have similar caloric values. A body of evidence is developing that implicates fructose as a significant factor in this. Fiber content of one's diet is also important. Little attention was paid to fiber content for a long time, probably because it does not contribute directly to the energy budget. It has become evident that the caloric and nutrient density of foods is an important factor in the development of diabetes. Obesity is a major risk factor for diabetes. The metabolic interactions of excess glucose, insulin, and lipid metabolism are complex and generally beyond the scope of this discussion. These interactions, when out of control tend to develop into a downward spiral, ultimately leading to disaster. We will focus on only a few of these interactions, which directly relate to our topic.

A Case History: The Pima Indians

The experience of the Pima Indians presents a natural experiment that illustrates the importance of lifestyle factors such as diet composition and exercise. The Pima Indians have lived in what is now the southwestern United States and northern Mexico for several thousand years. A major settlement is near the junction of the Gila and Salt Rivers in Arizona. The Pima Indians lived as a hunter-gatherer culture with some subsistence level agriculture supported by a sophisticated system of irrigation, and by all accounts were a healthy community. This way of life was upset in the late 19th century when settlers upstream diverted most of the water from the rivers, leaving the Pima Indians unable to continue to grow their own food. At the point of starvation, they were forced to live on government reservations and subsist on government-supplied food.

This new diet contained much more fat, sugar, and white flour than they had previously eaten. It is estimated that in 1890, their diet was composed of only 15 percent fat, but a mere thirty years later, fat composed 40 percent or more of their caloric intake. Their diet contained much more sugar and they engaged in much less physical activity. The incidence of obesity, diabetes, and its complications skyrocketed. Approximately half of adult Pima Indians now have diabetes. The Department of Indian Affairs and the U.S. Public Health Service have been conducting research studies on these problems as well as the genetics of the population. When they are able to reverse these lifestyle changes, the diabetes is at least partially controlled and the complications are reduced.

Yet the Pima Indians living in Mexico were spared this medical disaster. Although they are from the same genetic pool, they did not experience these problems at the same time as their northern counterparts. Other societies have demonstrated similar changes with the change in their diets, despite genetic similarity.

Increasing Accessibility of Sugar and Resultant Effects

According to Gary Taubes, as early as 1925, Haven Emerson, director of the Institute of Health at Columbia University, published a report with the observation that diabetes related deaths had increased fifteen fold in New York City since the Civil War, paralleling the increased consumption of sugar. Due to the lack of understanding of the metabolism of sugar and conflicting and erroneous information, the scientific community did not follow up on this observation.

After World War II, there was a great change in food preparation due to a gradual shift to a two-income household. With the wife working outside of the home, convenience became more important. More foods were prepared in a factory instead of at home. In the home, boxes of mixes replaced cooking from scratch, and the fast food industry began to flourish. The soft drink industry advertised heavily and their products became very popular, especially among adolescents. Industries increased the size of their containers repeatedly. The development of sports drinks and energy drinks further increased the consumption of sugar and high fructose corn syrup. In parallel, the rates of obesity and diabetes also increased.

For thousands of years, sugar was a minor part of the human diet. When sugar was present, it was composed of complex carbohydrates and mixed with fiber. This changed when the industrial revolution made it possible to refine sugar from sugar cane and later sugar beets. Initially, sugar was quite expensive and in many wealthy households was kept under lock and key. As the efficiency of the refining process was improved, the price decreased and sugar became increasingly affordable for more members of the rapidly expanding population. While accurate data sufficient for sophisticated statistical analysis is not available, this increase in access to sugar seems to parallel the divergence in health levels between the industrialized communities and the communities that continued on the diets of their ancestors. These observations, in various forms, by many different scientists, have been made for decades. Of course, association and correlation do not prove cause and effect, but they may be pieces of the puzzle. And the repetition of this pattern in many different cultures and situations is certainly suggestive of a relationship.

The label "sugar" has several meanings. Probably the most common usage refers to sucrose, the product of cane or sugar beet extraction. Chemically, sucrose is a molecule made up of a combination of glucose and fructose molecules. When the discussion is about blood sugar, the reference is to glucose. Glucose is the essential sugar for all higher animal metabolism; the body cannot function without glucose. There are a large number of other similar molecules that are chemically referred to as sugars, such as lactose, laevulose, maltose, pentose, sucralose, etc. Glucose and fructose are the focus for this discussion.

Processed Food Issues:
High Fructose Corn Syrup

High fructose corn syrup (HFCS) became available in the 1970s. The consumption of HFCS in the US increased from less than one pound per person per year in 1970 to 63.8 pounds per person per year in 2000. After some negative publicity, it decreased to 48.9 pounds per person per year in 2010. HFCS is sweeter and cheaper than cane sugar, and thus more desirable from the manufacturer's perspective.

However, because HFCS has a greater percentage of fructose, it has a more severe negative effect on long term health. Since the effects of fructose are now better understood, it can be argued that it meets the definition of a chronic poison and an addictive substance. Fructose must be metabolized in the liver, because other organs of the body are unable to use it. It is metabolized in the liver in a manner similar to how ethanol is metabolized, rather than through the metabolic pathways used for glucose and most other sugars. This leads to fatty deposits in the liver, and insulin resistance. Fructose does not stimulate the secretion of the hormone that signals "I am full now" to the brain, but it does stimulate the production of very low density lipoprotein (VLDL) cholesterol and triglycerides, both of which increase the risk of atherosclerosis (artery hardening).

HFCS does not meet the current Food and Drug Administration (FDA) requirements for safety of a food additive. It has been grandfathered into the "generally recognized as safe" (GRAS) category of food additives, partly for political reasons. The FDA has no plans to change this decision in the foreseeable future, according to Dr. Robert Lustig (pediatric endocrinologist at the University of California, San Francisco, and author of the book *Fat Chance*). Lustig is one of several health professionals currently writing about fructose and other GRAS list substances under fire for their potential contribution to diabetes and unhealthy weight gain.

With the introduction of HFCS and other processed foods into their diets, people began eating less fiber. The beneficial effects of fiber are often overlooked because it does not directly contribute to the energy budget of the body, but it may be regarded as an essential nutrient. Fiber slows the absorption of carbohydrates and reduces the stress on overtaxed endocrine regulation mechanisms.

One reason the Western diet gradually became more concentrated in calories and poor in nutrients is that managers of the food industry were naturally more focused on profits and increasing sales than on health. Market incentives were, and still are, skewed towards an unhealthy diet, leading to obesity, diabetes and its complications. Although the public health and nutrition communities are becoming aware of these problems, it is difficult to apply these lessons to specific geographic locations such as Appalachia, where we seem to be voluntarily repeating the Pima Indian experience on a larger scale. This is a nationwide problem, yet those places with limited food access and few choices for shopping, eating out, and growing one's own produce — in other words, rural and urban lower-income communities — suffer more. While the problem arguably stems from the food industry and a failure to regulate processed foods in the United States, it flows disproportionately to communities where these are the most accessible foods, be that by cost or availability.

A look at previous encounters between public health efforts to change the status quo and cultural forces resisting change may be enlightening in terms of how foods enter our daily diet without too much regulation or observation — or even with a genuine belief that they will be good for us, which turns out later to be debatable.

Processed Food Issues: Some Historic Examples

Several hundred years ago, white flour was determined to spoil more slowly during storage than whole wheat flour. In the 1920s, with the discovery of vitamins and vitamin deficiency diseases, research focused on the composition of the wheat kernel and the distribution of nutrient components. When it became apparent that removing the husk and endosperm to increase shelf life left the white flour deficient in important vitamins, efforts were directed towards remedying the problem. In 1942, the federal government announced that it would purchase only enriched flour for feeding the military. This had a rallying knock-on effect for the general public, and enriched flour became the predominant form available. In essence, enriched flour has natural nutrients taken out to preserve longevity, then vitamins added artificially to replace them.

Iodine is a trace element that is a necessary component of thyroid hormones. The availability of iodine in nature varies considerably geographically. In areas where the iodine content of the soil was very low, goiters and hypothyroidism was high. It was discovered that this could be reversed or prevented by the addition of small amounts of iodine to the diet. Since essentially all of the communities in the area needed iodine, the cheapest, most efficient way to provide it was by the addition to an abundant food. The salt industry was cooperative and the transition was made in the US without much difficulty. It remains a problem in India where the salt industry is diffuse and economies of scale are not available to the small salt merchants.

Vitamin D is present in many foods and is synthesized by the body if the body has sufficient exposure to sunlight. Vitamin D deficiency was identified as the cause of rickets in the early part of the twentieth century. In the 1930s, the dairy industry voluntarily began to add vitamin D to milk and many dairy products. The FDA requires that Vitamin D also be added to infant formula.

In the early decades of the twentieth century, observational studies identified a relationship between fluoride and tooth decay. In 1950, the results of controlled clinical trials were published and the effort to provide fluoride to the general population began, mostly by adding fluoride to municipal water supplies, although Switzerland chose to add it to salt. The U.S. Public Health Service issued guidelines and strongly encouraged the fluoridation process, but no federal laws were passed. Some localities adopted fluoridation quietly without controversy, while others had vigorous political fights between the proponents and those who opposed the addition on various grounds. Approximately 60–65 percent of the U.S. population now benefit from the fluoridation of drinking water.

Tobacco

Efforts to reduce the use of tobacco date back to 1604, when King James I of England wrote a treatise on the harmful effects of smoking and authorized a heavy tax on the importation of tobacco. It seems likely that he was disappointed in the results of his efforts.

In modern times, organized public education programs have been around for at least 60 years. Scientific studies linking tobacco use with cancer, heart disease, and chronic lung disease helped boost the effect of the educational campaigns. Government involvement was initially instigated by public sentiment. Public sentiment was mixed due to the relatively high percentage of smokers in the population. Congress and state legislatures were lobbied heavily. Governmental strategies at first were focused on taxation, education, regulation of advertising and warning labels on packaging.

There were a number of private lawsuits seeking damages due to impaired health and deaths. The tobacco companies fought these suits with every means possible. Probably the most successful lawsuits were filed by a consortium of states based on the health care costs attributable to tobacco usage by Medicaid recipients. Many locales were successful in passing regulations restricting smoking in public places, based on the evidence of the harmful effects of second hand smoke. The tobacco industry spent huge sums of money fighting government effort. They lobbied vigorously and advertised heavily. They encouraged any research that countered the public health position and questioned the research and tried to sow doubt in the public understanding of the problem. In addition to the potent addiction of nicotine, political forces fueled by the profitability of the tobacco industry and the number of people employed in tobacco production worked to counter governmental involvement. Sometimes setbacks occurred for reasons not directly related to the problem or industry efforts. In 2003, the Supreme Court declared a state law prohibiting tobacco advertisements near schools to be unconstitutional. Tobacco consumption in the U.S. dropped from 42 percent in the adult population in 1965 to 20.8 percent in 2006, a significant reduction, but still a significant problem.

Diabetes' Impact on the Appalachian Region

Diabetes has had a particularly significant impact on the Appalachian region. This area has been widely affected and the prevalence of diabetes continues to rise. Appalachia is a 205,000 square mile region involving 13 states, which follows the Appalachian Mountains from New York to Mississippi. Twenty-four million people live in Appalachia. Much of the region is rural; 42 percent of Appalachia's residents live in rural areas compared to 20 percent in the United States. This region has historically been marginalized compared to the rest of the nation, experiencing a greater degree of hardship, poverty and chronic disease than most other areas in the United States. The Appalachian region has long been characterized as an area and people differing from the rest of America in terms of geography, culture, and economy (Coyne, Demian-Popescu, and Friend 2006).

The Centers for Disease Control and Prevention (CDC) is responsible for monitoring the number of people with diabetes in the country. One way this is measured is through the Behavioral Risk Factor Surveillance System (BRFSS) which gathers data on diabetes prevalence (the number of disease cases in the population at any given time). The latest BRFSS report indicates that 10 percent of Appalachia is diabetic compared to 8 percent of the rest of the country. Because BRFSS data is self-reported, and some individuals may not be aware of their diabetes status, it is expected that the true rates of diabetes in this region are even higher than 10 percent.

The higher than average rates of diabetes and two of its major risk factors — namely obesity and physical inactivity — can be visualized with

CDC's county-level prevalence maps, available through CDC's website. These maps are generated using data from BRFSS. Counties with the highest percentage of adults with diabetes are generally clustered in the southeastern United States, encompassing much of central and southern Appalachia. This area is increasingly referred to as the "diabetes belt," as it takes the shape of a belt across this region of the country.

Roughly 30 percent of individuals who reside in counties within the diabetes belt live sedentary lifestyles compared to 25 percent of individuals who reside in counties outside of the diabetes belt. Similarly, 33 percent of individuals residing in counties within the diabetes belt were obese compared to 26 percent nationwide. BRFSS data helps to illustrate the change in diabetes rates in our country over time, revealing the startling growth in this disease within the last century. The growth of obesity and sedentary behaviors has coincided with this upward shift, suggesting widespread adoption of unhealthy lifestyle choices across the country. Appalachia has consistently emerged within this larger framework as a high-risk region for diabetes and its risk factors.

Fortunately, many of the risks for diabetes can be targeted with improved lifestyle habits; eating a high-fiber, low-calorie diet; increasing physical activity; and accessing regular, preventative health care. There lies a recurring problem specific to the Appalachian region when one discusses health care access and dietary choices: poverty.

The Intertwining of Poverty, Education and Poor Health

In 2008, 18 percent of Appalachian residents were considered impoverished. The Appalachian Regional Commission has identified 98 Appalachian counties as distressed due to their high levels of poverty and unemployment (arc.gov). According to a recent report by Barker and colleagues (2010) residents of distressed Appalachian counties are 33 percent more likely to report having diabetes than residents of non–Appalachian counties.

Poverty's influence on poor health in general varies, with some issues thoroughly researched, others suggested by association but not causal factors. Often, poverty translates into limited formal education, lack of quality health care, poor infrastructure (badly maintained roads, etc.). Lower income individuals and people from underserved areas are more likely to have unhealthy physical activity and dietary behaviors.

While it would seem intuitive that being poor would result in less food being eaten, and therefore a lower body mass index, most of the cheap, readily available foods in the United States are low in nutrients and high in calories, fat, and sugar. People with less money often consume more caloric foods than wealthier people because that is what is available to them. Overweight and obesity are closely linked to nutrition, and particularly low fruit and vegetable consumption. Unfortunately, processed foods are typically more affordable than healthy, fresh foods, such as fruits and vegetables. In rural Appalachian communities, the limited availability of grocery stores selling fresh produce may exacerbate this problem. Often, convenience stores sell highly processed foods, soft drinks full of sugars, and other options that contribute to obesity.

The geographic and economic isolation of many Appalachian regions in the era of increasing processed foods consumption has begun to show long-term consequences on resident's health (Swanson, Schoenberg, Davis, Wright, & Dollarhide 2012). A study by Swanson et al., (2012) found that the most commonly cited barriers to fruit and vegetable consumption and overall healthy diets were costs, convenience, and taste preference.

Food security as defined by the World Food Summit is having access at all times to sufficient, safe, nutritious food to maintain a healthy and active life. In general, individuals living in rural areas experience more food insecurity than those living in non-rural areas. Food insecurity is often associated with lower consumption of fruits and vegetables, and to unhealthy diets (Holben & Pheley 2006). In addition, studies have also found that individuals diagnosed with diabetes were significantly more likely to live in food-insecure households. Individuals from food-insecure households have higher BMIs and rates of obesity than those living in food-secure households (Holben & Pheley 2006). Because of the economic constraints placed on those living in Appalachia, many households subsist on cheap, processed foods, which may in part explain the higher rates of diabetes seen in these areas because obesity and diabetes are so closely linked.

Physical activity and nutrition often go hand-in-hand when attempting to prevent obesity and diabetes. Engaging in regular physical activity is one of the most important lifestyle behaviors that one can perform in order to reduce the risk of obesity and its linked diseases. Because people in Appalachia's distressed counties are more likely to be eating cheaper, processed foods, they have an increased risk for developing obesity, cardiovascular disease, and cancer. Yet Appalachian residents are considered being the most sedentary population in the nation (Hortz, Stevens, Holden, & Petosa 2009). A study that looked at the rates of physical activity among Appalachian adolescents in Ohio found that only 5 percent of adolescents were engaging in the recommended amount of physical activity. Only 14 percent reported engaging in vigorous activity at least three days a week (Hortz et al., 2009). Overall, adolescents residing in Appalachia reported rates of physical activity well below recommended and national levels.

While ability to purchase healthy foods may stem from circumstances outside the control of an individual or family, how can decisions about physical activity be anything other than the responsibility of those same individuals or families? And yet, there are several environmental causal factors documented for lack of physical activity in adolescents, including transportation, tight school budgets, and work/chores (Hortz et al., 2009).

Because school districts often cover vast geographic regions, providing bus transportation between school and home is often an issue. In addition, tight school budgets limit the number of after school programs that schools can offer. Lastly, many adolescents are required to work after school or have chores that they are expected to perform at home. While these duties could be physically demanding, they may also be less exercise than is needed on a daily basis. Add to these the limited accessibility of safe places in which to exercise (sidewalks, lighted pathways, gymnasiums, swimming pools with cheap access, etc.) and these factors together may limit the amount of physical activity options, not just for adolescents, but for most rural Appalachians.

Adults residing in Appalachia also report lower rates of physical activity. In Kentucky, as one example, 24 percent of adults reported being inactive, meaning less than ten minutes of physical activity per week (Kruger, Swanson, Davis, Wright, Dollarhide, & Schoenberg, 2012). There are multiple barriers to engaging in physical activity that adults in this region report experiencing including: responsibilities at home, transportation issues, lack of access to appropriate facilities, inadequate programming and activities, and poor weather. Participants in focus groups conducted by Kruger et al., often reported that they felt guilty taking time away from their family and other responsibilities to engage in physical activity. Additionally, living in a rural area often requires residents to travel long distances to reach common destinations such as, work, schools, and grocery stores, resulting in much of their discretionary time being spent traveling. Living in a rural area also affects what facilities or programs are available to the community. Often, state-sponsored recreational facilities and programs are too far away for residents to attend. Private facilities may be limited to certain residents by fee or membership, with the result that some residents may not be able to access them. Other fitness businesses may open in rural areas, only to find too few subscribing members for the population base to justify their equipment costs.

Poverty and education are often strongly correlated. Studies of perceptions and knowledge related to diabetes in Appalachia highlight a lack of understanding of the risk factors for diabetes. Lower levels of educational attainment in Appalachia may contribute to inadequate prevention and treatment of diabetes. For example, individuals may not know that a lack of physical activity and poor dietary behaviors can ultimately lead to diabetes. Many of the risks for diabetes, such as tobacco use and weight management, are modifiable; therefore, education about how individuals can avoid these risks is necessary for lowering the prevalence of diabetes in Appalachia (Denham et al., 2010). A study conducted by Tessaro, Smith, and Rye (2005), found that among the Appalachian population there is a general lack of knowledge about diabetes, even after diagnosis. They also found that a lot of blame and guilt are associated with the diagnosis of diabetes because it is felt that it is a self-induced disease that is caused by a general laziness and lack of self-discipline. These feeling are associated with awareness the community self-reports regarding the lack of physical activity and diets high in sugar and fat often seen in this region.

A common misconception is that diabetes is caused by heredity and only strikes every other generation (Tessaro et al., 2005). Several barriers to early detection of diabetes were identified through the study. Two major barriers were the inability to recognize the symptoms of diabetes, and not having a regular health care provider.

Diabetes care depends on a combination of access to quality health care and proper self-management. Access to health care is a barrier experienced by many residents of Appalachia. In this region, many people do not seek preventative care because of the high costs or far distances. It has been noted that, even if an individual is experiencing health issues or symptoms they will often neglect to inform their health care provider for fear that medications will be prescribed or tests ordered for which they cannot pay. Transportation issues were also cited as a major health care barrier; because much of the region is rural and provider shortages are widespread it is often necessary for residents to travel up to an hour away to receive proper care.

The United States Department of Health and Human Services has deemed many areas of Appalachia "health professional shortage areas" or "medically underserved areas." These labels indicate the struggle many residents of Appalachia face to accessing adequate health care and education about diabetes prevention and self-management. Efforts to recruit physicians and primary medical providers to the region are ongoing.

Potential Solutions

A growing number of health education initiatives in the region aim to increase awareness of diabetes risks and teach individuals and communities how they can prevent diabetes and/or improve diabetic care. A combination of population health programs, policies, and individualized treatment are important for a comprehensive diabetes prevention strategy.

One good example of a collaborative effort to address diabetes in the region is the Appalachian Diabetes Control and Translation Project. In 2000, the Centers for Disease Control and Prevention (CDC) partnered with the Appalachian Regional Commission (ARC), the Robert C Byrd Center for Rural Health at Marshall University, and states across Appalachia to implement the project. This effort builds on federal, state and community partnerships to: establish policies that prevent diabetes and improve related health outcomes; develop diabetes prevention programs using evidence based education resources (e.g., "Diabetes Today" by the CDC); and collect data on diabetes prevalence in the region. As of 2011, some 74 diabetes coalitions had been established in economically distressed counties in 9 Appalachian states. Coalition projects varied in scope to include education on healthy eating and physical activity, health fairs, health support groups, and other programs that do not involve direct clinical care.

The coalitions also offer training in, among other topics, diabetes self-management. In 2008 alone, individuals in Appalachia were involved in coalition community health projects 52,842 times (number of encounters) while 1,372 individuals were trained in chronic disease self-management or diabetes care.

The introduction of policies to increase access to healthy foods in Appalachia may help curb the obesity and diabetes rates. At the federal level, policies to reduce subsidies of corn and soy and associated cheap sources of sugar and fat could reduce the presence of highly processed foods available for consumers. Sugar and fat taxes to generate revenue for healthy food programs have also been proposed at state levels. At the community level, healthy school lunch programs, such as Farm to School, may provide more fresh food options. Community based interventions, including cooking classes and diabetes education workshops, could provide individuals with skills to prepare fresh, healthy foods and the knowledge to make choices to prevent obesity and diabetes. While this does not address the ability to procure such foods economically, it does start down a road worth traveling.

Educational initiatives and other public health programs should build on Appalachia's unique cultural features. Many scholars and journalists throughout history have stereotyped the residents of Appalachia as being uneducated fundamentalists who are culturally homogenous and live in isolation from the rest of the country. Focus groups conducted by Coyne et al., however, found that the aforementioned attributes do not adequately describe the residents of Appalachia.

As one example, individuals residing in West Virginia characterized themselves as kind, outgoing, helpful, and with a strong work ethic. Participants of the focus groups were proud to be from Appalachia and to be able to call the mountains their home. They felt that their strongest qualities were an abiding faith in God, family values, and solid morals (Coyne et al., 2006). Participants in this study objected to the media portrayal of what being "Appalachian" meant. They felt that the stereotypical view of Appalachia did not describe them at all, and were often offended by the media's characterization of them as uneducated, poverty-laden people.

This rejection of being considered impoverished adds a layer of complexity to dealing with issues of poverty in Appalachia, which by the ARC's definition has no fewer than 96 distressed counties. The effects of poverty on health, particularly diabetes, have been focused on in this essay at length. A people group that refutes a poverty stereotype, but which exemplifies the effects of poverty on its health, must be handled with cultural empathy and understanding. Perhaps the concern of those who consider themselves stereotyped is less that poverty is prevalent in Appalachia, than how that poverty has been portrayed as a blanket condemnation. As one participant stated, "We haven't been individualized; we have been categorized."

Appalachia has many deep-seated traditions and cultural values, and effective programs will need to recognize these cultural differences while not holding back on mitigating barriers to healthy living. Again, cultural sensitivity and a good listening ear will be required. As one example, existing stereotypes portray traditional family structure in Appalachia as the wife being the homemaker and the husband as the head of the household. As with the rest of the world, Appalachia has faced economic strains with resultant changes in social roles. As in many families, where employment is available it is likely that both parents are in the workforce. Also, studies show that when decisions about medical care/treatment need to be made, women are the gatekeepers and appointment makers regarding family health, and men act in accordance with their directives (Welch 2011).

And yet, while there may have been many shifts in family roles, family cohesion still plays a strong role in the lives of people from Appalachia (Coyne et al., 2006). Large, close knit extended families are very common in most communities throughout Appalachia, and this sense of family provides strong social support. At the same time, it is important to note that it is often felt that "family problems" are to remain in the family and not be discussed with anyone outside of the immediate or extended family. This characteristic is important because the taboo includes seeking care and support from medical facilities. Seeking help from a medical facility is usually viewed as a last resort. Earlier discussion centered on economic, geographic or educational barriers to accessing medical care. Now a fourth can be identified: cultural taboos. A general distrust of medical care providers from outside the area continues to exist, and this can be laid at the feet of cultural differences. It has also been reported that participants find it hard to build trustful relationships with providers due to high turnover rates, as some residents take positions in rural areas as part of a debt forgiveness program, or to obtain American visas in the case of foreign-born professionals. The high turnover rate has been found to be a deterrent to seeking health care (Coyne et al., 2006).

As Yogi Berra has been quoted "making predictions is difficult, especially about the future." We have looked at the problem of diabetes in Appalachia but what does it all mean? However, we think that there are some lessons to be learned. We have identified some of the biological factors that lead to the development of diabetes, and explored some of the cultural, sociological and political details that influence these factors. Of all the influences cited, it would be difficult to point to any single factor and call it unique to Appalachia. Other regions have been sparsely populated, isolated, difficult to navigate, poor, low in educational attainment, suspicious of outsiders, and lacking in health food stores. Some regions combine several of these factors. Is Appalachia the only region that combines all of them? Perhaps not; to quote a cliché, "the jury is still out."

But the fact remains that Appalachia does have all of these factors working against the health and wellbeing of its residents. Guiding change into constructive directions is difficult, and cannot be effected long-term by those outside the region without leadership and partnership from those within it.

There are many cross currents, some large and some small, that influence changes. Money is critical to diabetes prevention and control. The impoverished individual is handicapped in his efforts to deal with both diabetes risk factors (prevention) and diabetes itself (control). Similarly, community efforts are blunted by inadequate financial resources, and the economic recession has only aggravated the problem. Vested interests that profit from either the status quo or negative influences can be expected to resist change. Nutrition contents in processed foods, the inclusion of substances such as high fructose corn syrup, and the exclusion of sugary soft drinks from "adolescent zones" such as schools could be described, in today's realities, as being handled as political decisions driven by market forces more so than health decisions. Education is important from both an individual and community perspective. It is important for an individual to learn how to take care of themselves. Education at the community level is necessary for constructive public policy development. But it must be respectful to and based in the cultural values and expectations of that community, or it will neither take effect nor stick.

A personal anecdote may lend perspective to this problem of building solutions from within the community instead of imposing them from without. The high school from which Dr. Carl Greever, one of this essay's authors, graduated six decades ago eventually merged with several other high schools in the same county as population declined, moving from local governance to county. In 2001, the state board of education took over the administration of the county schools, citing an inability of the county board to maintain standards. Now community reports in print and conversation bemoan the fact that the state has itself had little success. As one example, a number of positions that stayed vacant for several years without the board receiving any applications. Additionally, out of seven high school class reunions, only the first two were held in the community, because after that time there were no local facilities deemed adequate for the reunion. Population continued to decline, taking with it the economic prosperity the community had once enjoyed.

Such population decline, and the shifting of decision-making from local to state, is more common in rural Appalachian than urban. And certainly there are brighter spots in some parts of rural Appalachia than the community above, but its story is representative of a very large problem. And as population declines, dragging economic development and sustainable community life behind it, the struggle for improvement faces a very steep slope.

On a brighter note, informal educational efforts are having some effect. Some schools are successfully removing junk foods and beverages from vending machines in county or town decision-making. There are efforts to provide better choices in school cafeterias and to educate students about good nutrition choices. Productions of both sugar and HFCS have decreased for the last several years and foods labeled HFCS-free are appearing in the market place, largely due to popular demand from consumer pressures. As just one example, Morgan Spurlock (a native of Appalachia) won first prize at the Sundance Film Festival for his documentary film, "Supersize Me" and McDonald's subsequently dropped the promotion of "supersizing" meals from their menu. Manufacturers are becoming increasingly aware that a significant portion of the target population has a negative opinion of HFCS.

More research on nutrition would be helpful to provide guidance and motivation. There is little to no funding available in the present economic climate. The natural history of disease is significant. People are developing diabetes at earlier ages than previous generations. Once diabetes has developed in an individual, it and its complications are difficult to reverse even in ideal conditions. Unfortunately for many in Appalachia, the conditions are far from ideal. This spells great difficulties for a community in both personal burden of disease, costs due to patient care, lost productivity, and consequently tax contribution to the community. In essence, rural Appalachia is not sparsely populated, but those who live there are becoming increasingly unhealthy.

The prevalence of diabetes will remain high until significant changes come into the dietary and physical activity behaviors of individuals residing in Appalachia. These changes can best be made within individual communities, supported by federal efforts such as HFCS being removed from the GRAS list, and state grants for local initiatives such as "Diabetes Today." Changes of this kind may be best measured in generations rather than years.

References

Centers for Disease Control and Prevention: National Diabetes Surveillance System. http://apps.nccd.cdc.gov/DDTSTRS/default.aspx (accessed 27 February 2012).

Coyne, C.A., Demian-Popescu, C., and Friend, D. 2006. "Social and Cultural Factors Influencing Health in Southern West Virginia: A Qualitative Study." *Preventing Chronic Disease* 3 (4): A124.

Crespo et al., 2011. "Appalachian Regional Model for Organizing and Sustaining County-Level Diabetes Coalitions." *Health Promotion and Practice* 12 (4): 544–550.

Denham S.A., Wood L.E., and Remsberg, K. 2010. "Diabetes Care: Provider Disparities in the US Appalachian Region." *Rural and Remote Health* 10: 1320. http://www.rrh.org.au.

Holben, D.H., and Pheley, A.M. 2006. "Diabetes Risk and Obesity in Food-insecure Households in Rural Appalachian Ohio." *Preventing Chronic Disease* 3 (3): A82.

Kruger, T.M., Swanson, M., Davis, R.E., Wright, S., Dollarhide, K., and Schoenberg, N.E. 2012. "Formative Research Conducted in Rural Appalachia to Inform a Community Physical Activity." *American Journal of Health Promotion: AJHP* 26 (3), 143–151. doi:10.4278/ajhp.091223-QUAL-399

Lustig, Robert H. et, al. 2012. "The Toxic Truth about Sugar." *Nature* 482 (2 February): 27–29.

Quinn, Samantha. 2012. *The Real Truth about Sugar: Dr. Robert Lustig's Sugar, the Bitter Truth.* Doylestown, PA: River City eBooks.

Spurlock, Morgan. 2005. *Don't Eat This Book.* New York: The Penguin Group.

Swanson, M., Schoenberg, N.E., Davis, R., Wright, S., and Dollarhide, K. 2012. "Perceptions of Healthful Eating and Influences on the Food Choices of Appalachian Youth." *Journal of Nutrition Education and Behavior,* doi:10.1016/j.jneb.2011.07.006.

Taubes, Gary. 2007. *Good Calories, Bad Calories.* New York: Anchor.

Taubes, Gary. 2011. *Why We Get Fat and What to Do About It.* New York: Alfred A. Knopf.

Tessaro, I., Smith, S.L., and Rye, S. 2005. "Knowledge and Perceptions of Diabetes in an Appalachian Population." *Preventing Chronic Disease* 2 (2): A13.

Welch, Wendy. 2011. "Self-Control, Fatalism and Health in Appalachia." *Journal of Appalachian Studies* Vol. 17, Issue 1/2: 108.

Williams, K.J., Taylor, C.A., Wolf, K.N., Lawson, R.F., and Crespo, R. 2008. "Cultural Perceptions of Healthy Weight in Rural Appalachian Youth." *Rural and Remote Health* 8 (2): 932.

Yudkin, John. 1972. *Pure White and Dangerous.* London: Viking.

When OxyContin Struck, and How the Community Struck Back: One Woman Remembers

SUE ELLA KOBAK

The last time I saw Little Paul alive, he was halfway under his trailer trying to fix his water line. It was mid–August 2008 and his dad was nearby "supervising." Little Paul ducked his head out and gave me a smile, reminding me he was his father's son. Just a few weeks later, my husband and I attended his funeral.

On that warm September evening — a night too beautiful to mark such a sad occasion — the church was packed. My first impression on arriving was, how are they going to park this many cars in that tiny church lot safely? Art and I parked on the side of a narrow road, already lined by cars doing the same.

Poor Bottom — the name of the place and the Free Will Baptist church in question — now has black asphalt roads, but during my youth, they were dirt and gravel. Many of the friends who went to Poor Bottom's one room elementary school with me were at the funeral. Some had left home after high school to get jobs or join the military, and many had returned in their retirement years to become active members of the community; others had stayed and made lives in the area, never leaving.

Sitting in the church that day, attending the funeral of a boy just a third of our age, it would have been hard to know which were which. Cousins, uncles, aunts, friends, neighbors: the holler community was there. We all said hello and hugged each other.

Little Paul, the son of dear friends, was 27 when he died. He'd been addicted to prescription drugs since his teen years. There he lay in his ball cap, his jeans and shirt, dead from a self-inflicted bullet wound to the head. At least, that was the official write-up by the authorities, but we all knew that his drug addiction really had done the job.

He had recently gone to a doctor's office in Williamson, West Virginia, where he received a prescription for 60 Xanax and 60 Lorcets. He told friends he'd paid the doctor $375 for the visit and that she never drew blood or took any vital information.

None of us know exactly when he went back again, just that it was some time in late August; he got prescriptions for additional drugs. Before his death he had taken them all: the 60 Xanax, the 60 Lortab, and the new prescriptions. He was clean out of drugs when he died.

At the funeral, anger burned against the doctor who wrote those prescriptions; stories ran through the church crowd about the line of people in her office, all the way out the door and down the street. "She should be put out of business, but the drug enforcement forces get rid of one greedy pill pusher and another pops up. You can't win."

It was a hot day and still very warm as the evening services started. The church was without air conditioning, but fans moved and windows stood open. The air hung heavy like the sadness in the room.

My husband, Art Van Zee, and I approached the parents, Paul and Carol, with such a sense of pain for their loss. Paul is a strong person. He grew up poor, very poor. He worked hard in the coal mines until multiple back injuries put him out on insurance compensation.

He will never work as a coal miner again, but Paul is not somebody who can be idle. He slowly, an hour here and an hour there, hiring help when he could afford it, began building his and Carol's dream home.

Carol too has always been a hard worker; her job as a certified nurses' assistant in a local nursing home is hard work, but she does it well and with a caring attitude. They truly are good people.

The singing started. Expressive voices conveyed loss and hopelessness, yet also belief in the loving nature of a just and good God. That seemed the only hope left in the room. The Reverend Richard spoke about a loving and forgiving God, and you could have heard the proverbial pin drop. Everybody knew about the sin of suicide, but wanted the preacher to offer some hope; he did.

"It's times like this when a minister spends a great deal of time reading through the Bible, asking for direction and inspiration," he began, wiping his forehead with a handkerchief.

His message told us that we were not the ones to judge, that the good lord was a merciful God, that theology teaches us to hope that we will receive eternal life through the redemption of Jesus. His words gave the condolence

Little Paul's family needed — and the parents, neighbors and friends sat listening, wondering whose child would be next.

At the end of his sermon, the Reverend Richard said the congregation would provide a meal for the family at 3 p.m. the next day. He added a strange coda to this announcement: that he was aware that members of the congregation "had already been through this recently," and he understood if some families "couldn't do it again, for financial or emotional reasons, either one."

After the services, friends informed me that the day before they had buried another victim. A young boy — who should have been a man, except for the arresting effects of addiction — died in a fire on the hill where he lived in a camper trailer. He was a heavy drug user.

Nobody knew exactly what happened, but the prevailing view was that he'd been too high to get himself out when the fire started. It probably started by him smoking in bed, or lighting the gas stove ring.

Little Paul was good friends with one of my relatives and I already knew that they had shared Xanax and marijuana the morning Little Paul died. At the funeral, he held me tight and tried to reassure me that he was doing well with his drug problem and hadn't used in two months. But all of us felt, on leaving the church house, that we could soon be the next grieving family. There are very few families in the coal fields that have not been affected directly or indirectly by a prescription drug problem.

The emotional struggle of the day lingered for some time. Feelings of anger and frustration flooded me, watching a culture I treasured and belonged to slide into an unrecognizable tangle of trauma, terror and stereotypes. A strong sense that "it all has changed" pervaded that funeral, meaning the impact of prescription drug abuse has changed us all forever, and not for the better.

Many of us have worked so hard for years to try to confront the disease of addiction that has set about destroying central Appalachia. Art (a medical doctor) and I are among many in this fight. Art treats addicts as outpatients at the community health clinic, and in my career as a lawyer, I have often worked with offenders to find paths to rehabilitation rather than incarceration, to put the axe to the root of the tree rather than its branches, via drug courts and laws that targeted pharmaceutical companies. Those of us in this fight have long been aware that prescription drug abuse was a problem, but the introduction of OxyContin by Purdue Pharma hit all sectors of people, families, professionals, resources — hit them really hard, and really fast.

In looking back over forty years of fighting substance abuse, particularly prescription substance abuse, I think we did some things right, and

I think we missed a major opportunity. Below I will try to explore some of what's happened over the years, using Lee County, Virginia (where I now live and work) as an example.

The Beginnings of "The Epidemic"

Anecdotal evidence of "the epidemic" started spreading as early as 1999 in communities like Lee County, shortly after OxyContin (the drug's trade name) was introduced. OxyContin is one of the leading drugs for abuse, primarily because it was widely prescribed as a pain reliever in the late 1990s. Communities with higher rates of physical labor jobs — like coal mining — began to see fathers, brothers, sons, and yes, mothers, wives, and daughters, on this painkiller at a phenomenal rate.

OxyContin is a brand name of a preparation of oxycodone (an opioid) with a time release preparation. The drug provided convenience because it was taken twice daily. It was never shown to be more effective than short-acting oxycodone, taken four times daily. Purdue Pharma of Stamford, Connecticut, marketed the painkiller very aggressively, trivializing the risks, inferring there was very low addiction potential, and over-selling the benefits. The company was able to obtain the right, through the Food and Drug Administration (FDA) approval process, to allow the medication to be indicated for moderate to severe pain. Moderate pain can be medically defined as a high school football player getting a knee injured and being on crutches for six weeks, moderate chronic arthritic pain, or even having a tooth pulled. This resulted in the drug being more widely prescribed.

In 1999, Vince Stravino, a doctor practicing in Lee County, Virginia, began sharing stories about the drug and the overdose patients he was seeing with Art. Two nuns, Sisters Elizabeth Vines and Beth Davies, had already worked in the community for over thirty years providing addiction education; they, too, were hearing and seeing some of the impact of this drug from local people. Stravino personally called the FDA and the pharmaceutical company regarding the incidences he was seeing in 1999. After receiving little response from the FDA or the company regarding his concerns, Stravino turned to a second resource.

Lee County has many people who have experience in community organizing. Several years previously, people from local agencies, churches, health care professionals and the department of social services had created the Lee Coalition for Health (aka the Coalition). The Coalition is a not-for-profit Virginia corporation. As a group, they had been actively involved in improvement of the health of people in Lee County through education and sponsorship of community health events like cancer screenings, pre-natal care events, and smoking cessation campaigns.

Amid the rising tide of addiction and deaths associated with addic-tion, a significant amount of anecdotal information became more prevalent within the county, causing the Coalition to turn its focus toward problems of prescription drug addiction and abuse. Art obtained an assessment ques-tionnaire from the Center for Disease Control. It was designed to gather information about the various health habits of adolescents within a com-munity. He and other Coalition members went to the Lee County School Board to obtain permission to submit the questionnaire to all of the Lee County students in grades seven through twelve. The school board would not allow the questions that related to the sexual habits of the teens as part of the assessment, but let the rest of the questions stand.

The questionnaire was administered, collected, and turned over to the Coalition. Garrett Keys, a potential medical student, was employed through the East Tennessee Medical School Appalachian Summer program. Keys collated the questionnaire information, obtained volunteers to input the information into a database, and secured the use of the school computer labs and the support of the computer teachers in the county who worked as volunteers. It should be noted that students were involved in this process as often as possible. Kevin Carson, president of the Lee County High School student body, organized student volunteers who were supervised by the volunteer teachers while they did the data input. Someone in the commu-nity even provided pizzas for the crew. Because of the prior effectiveness of the Coalition, the community trusted the efforts being made.

After the data was computerized, Keys and my husband began the analysis. The pervasiveness of prescription drug abuse, particularly the drug OxyContin, were astounding. It appeared from the data that at least 9 percent of seventh graders and 24 percent of eleventh graders in Lee County had used OxyContin at least once.

Using OxyContin to get high requires only the ability to destroy the time release component by crushing or even chewing the tablet. Thus, OyxContin can be easily abused (Meier 2003). After the time release com-ponent is destroyed the user can swallow the powder, snort the drug or dissolve the powder in water and inject the drug intravenously. Either of these options gives an immediate, heroin-like high. Communities in the late 1990s were beginning to see overdose victims on a regular bases, pre-dominately teens and young adults.

As Art and I stood with Garrett in our kitchen, looking at the bars and graphs that he had prepared, Art said, "Remember that book by Claude Brown?"

It was as though he'd read my mind. Brown's autobiography, *A Man-child in a Promised Land*, talked about the impact on the culture and lives of black people in Harlem, New York, when heroin hit the inner city.

Even though this was an informal assessment, the questionnaire provided good information to support the stories (what some called, perhaps hopefully, "rumors") and would be helpful in designing a plan for addressing the problem. The Coalition and several other organizations began campaigns to educate and inform the public of the problem's scope and magnitude. At the same time, newspapers in northern Maine began describing the same problems. As mentioned earlier, OxyContin tended to be marketed aggressively to communities where heavy labor was prevalent. What these two areas had in common was the nature of physical labor in the coal fields and the logging industry. In central Appalachia many people have been physically injured in the coal mines, while in northern Maine a good number had physical injuries as a result of working in the logging industry. Thus physically injured people from both areas were taking various types of prescription pain medication — among them OxyContin. And its use was rising quickly, particularly in rural, labor-intensive regions.

Purdue Pharma

In preparation for OxyContin coming onto the market, Purdue Pharma acquired data banks of information that provided the prescribing habits of doctors from all across the country. Because the doctors in central Appalachia and northern Maine were treating a lot of people for moderate chronic pain, these areas hit their marketing radar very quickly. Purdue Pharma designed a marketing campaign using this data. Sales representatives were given information about the individual doctor's prescribing habits so they could target these doctors.

Purdue Pharma's marketing campaign involved "continuing educational programs." This meant that approximately 5,000 doctors and nurses were sent, all expenses paid, to 40 different conferences at various resorts in Florida, Arizona, and California. They received education related to what was presented as the growing problem of under-treated pain. Some doctors were trained to be trainers themselves and received monetary compensation for this work.

Research into the effects of pharmaceutical seminars and gifts (from beach hats to compact discs) shows an interesting dichotomy in medical thinking. Asked if such gifts or events influence their prescription decisions, doctors will most often say no, but that they think some other doctors are influenced. In 2000, Purdue Pharma spent over 200 million dollars on their marketing campaign to sell OxyContin. They also funded lay organizations that were advocating aggressive treatment of pain. Many of these projects did not say to the general public that they were being funded by Purdue Pharma; a little digging was required to find that information.

Thus, it appears that many doctors were influenced by the information given to them in a very effective marketing scheme. In both rural Maine and central Appalachia, doctors who were already heavy pain medication prescribers, often overworked and willing to take someone's word for it, relied on the sales representatives to give them valid information. Doctors received coupons that gave their patients a certain amount of OxyContin free, among other incentives. During a sales campaign that ended in 2000, more than 3,400 coupons had been redeemed nationally, each providing a free 7 to 30 day supply. Bonus incentives were paid to sales representatives for their aggressive sale of the drug.

In 1996 the sale of the drug was $48 million; by 2000 sales were almost $1.1 billion. In 2012, it topped $2.8 billion (Bourdet). Marketing efforts could be described as fairly successful.

The Community Response: Action, Fragmentation, Frustration

Lee County, like many Appalachian communities, has several people actively involved in community organization on a wide range of topics and levels. In the 1990s, many people in the county worked together to stop the efforts of private landfill development in Lee County; halt unregulated strip mining; and improve the region's water quality.

However, it became clear early on that the problem was much bigger than Lee County. The region and the nation were seeing the same things as Lee Countians. Appalachian Substance Abuse Coalition, a loose association of regional professional addiction and mental health workers, began to meet regarding the problem. Early on it became clear that the problem was wide-spread, and growing. Unfortunately, state-wide organizations that might have been able to work with this epidemic saw it primarily as a rural problem.

As one example, the Virginia Organizing Project (now "Virginia Organizing") is a not-for-profit corporation dedicated to education, support and organization within the Commonwealth of Virginia's communities. The first chapter of the VOP started in Lee County, so by the time the community began challenging OxyContin abuse, VOP had become established enough to employ a regional organizer: Jill Carson, who lived in Lee County. But, at that time, VOP did not work across state lines, respond to issues on an immediate basis, or see the need to organize groups of people from a wide range of socioeconomic backgrounds around this issue. The urban/rural divide was difficult; the rich/poor divide was nearly impossible.

Thus, most early responses to the OxyContin epidemic were based within specific communities. St. Charles Community Health Center was organized by the people of the community with the assistance of the Vanderbilt Student Health Coalition, which had hired Art in the late 1970s. (The clinic is now part of Stone Mountain Health Services, a group of clinics that has operated as a community owned health system for many years.)

But even as communities acted, larger organizations did not. The United Mine Workers of America has a long history of representing coal miners' holistic needs well in the entire southwestern part of Virginia. But again, OxyContin crossed economic and social lines, and it was also seen as something of a "medical" problem instead of a rampant issue affecting everyone. Meanwhile, local social services agencies, mental health agencies, law enforcement systems, and the legal system began to see addiction to OxyContin affect their budgets, pushing their staff to the limit, even harming people they worked with as fellow service providers. The crime rate for breaking and entering, as well as grand and petit larceny in Lee County and surrounding areas, was increasing exponentially. Other counties in southwestern Virginia, eastern Kentucky, and West Virginia were becoming increasingly aware of the dynamics involved with this prescription drug abuse. Federal enforcement agencies like the Tobacco and Fire Arms Control, the Federal Bureau of Investigation, and the United States Attorney's office began sounding the alarm on the resulting criminal problems from the addictive use of OxyContin.

As the federal agencies began to show interest, newspaper, magazines, television and other media attention started being given to this problem. "Hillbilly Heroin" became a common phrase to describe the situation. By now, however, the problem had spread well beyond northern Maine and the central Appalachian region. Negative stereotyping never helps, of course, and because the people of the region felt the impact and identified the problem early on, the perception of the problem continued to be that it affected Appalachia more than any other area. This continued marginalization of the problem echoes that of Harlem, and its reputation for drugs; like Harlem, central Appalachia became a rural ghetto with a mental border around it. Inside, a sign read: here are the addicts.

The twenty-first century rolled along while local law enforcement agencies and authorities began to investigate and prosecute doctors for illegal prescribing, as well as drug traffickers, and addicts who sold to support their own habit. Art contacted and met with several of Lee County's area agencies to share their perspectives on the problems; other community leaders around the region were doing the same. Thus, the community started to identify and address the problem at the same time. (From participating in those meetings, I can state categorically that, as one can imagine, the most sensitive group were parents, dealing with significant problems that they never imagined they would have to address. This group was in visible pain.)

Jails were filling up fast at both the federal and state level. As a part of this criminal activity, the Department of Social Services saw a significant increase in the numbers of children in their foster care program. OxyContin became the intergenerational scourge: grandparents, parents, children all felt its effects.

The first efforts of the Coalition included setting up a public forum at the high school auditorium, including law enforcement and education officials. Over eight hundred people attended, including many parents, preachers and church people, teachers, law enforcement professionals and medical or social workers who worked with addiction. They all had a vested interest in this problem. Out of this effort several focus groups formed to plan for action, as well as very active parent and family support groups. Sisters Beth and Elizabeth worked with family and friends, and with the loved ones in jail for drug-related offenses. The sisters held regular meetings for inmates at the county courthouse.

Even with this good start, it was soon clear that more was needed. The list included:

1. treatment for the people addicted
2. drug courts to help addicts get back into the community as contributing citizens
3. holding the drug companies accountable
4. major efforts into controlling the availability of the drug
5. and education regarding addiction for the general population.

As a result of the local Community Services Board, an agency that tried to take a multi-disciplinary approach, many agencies, individuals, and groups wanted to better understand the problem themselves and educate as many people as possible about what was happening. It was decided to develop an educational forum as soon as possible. All the groups pooled funds to obtain a location, a catered meal, and approval for accreditation from the relevant professional organizations (mental health, prescription providers, etc.). The resulting forum was a great success: widely attended, informative, useful for on-the-ground service providers, and an area-wide discussion of the problem involving the community. Thereafter several professional groups in Virginia, Kentucky, West Virginia, and Tennessee formed various efforts to discuss the problem region wide.

While this seemed a promising outcome of those early efforts, the unfortunate result was fragmentation of knowledge and power, and a scattering of resources into impractically small pieces. Working in their own States, everyone realized that OxyContin was a national problem, but turf, territory and resources were allocated, sought, sometimes even fought over on a community, state and regional level. I attended several of these meetings and conferences with my husband; watching and becoming increasing involved with both the grass roots and professional efforts of many good people desperate to help their communities, it became clear that the limited resources available to fight the drug's hold were being squandered in small, fragmented efforts, while the multi-national drug companies rolled on. Purdue Pharma needed to be confronted and held accountable on a federal level regarding the aggressive sales efforts which contributed to the drug being so readily available. By now, the drug sold for $1.00 per milligram on the streets and was easy to get.

A local nursing home in Dryden, Virginia, closed at about this time, and the 1970s building was given to the Lee County Coalition. In need of fundamental repairs to the plumbing, electric wiring, and roof, the property included more than four acres of land and was well situated for access, but also privacy. The Coalition met, and decided this was the perfect place to locate a residential treatment facility for addiction treatment. Now the community had a project that was concrete and designed to provide a service not available within a 100 mile radius. It took three years, a lot of sweat equity, help from the Job Corps, deals from local contractors, but New Beginnings in southwest Virginia opened its doors in November 2005 with the mission to provide long-term residential treatment to individuals from the region, regardless of their ability to pay. In the seven years it was open, more than 800 individuals received treatment. Sadly, New Beginnings closed in 2012. This was a great loss to the region and to many individuals who could have been well served by treatment there.

While support abounded within the grass roots community for a treatment facility, funds were not always forthcoming from other sources. Local economic development money was hard to find for the project. Lee County sits inside a three-county municipal district called LENOWISCO;

neither its director, nor the county Economic Development Authority director, nor the members of the Coalfield Economic Development Commission, considered addiction an economic issue—even as rumors that local coal companies were having trouble hiring sober miners turned to full-on newspaper stories, and to boardroom reports given back at headquarters.

At the time it was baffling to see a region coming apart at the seams deny it had a problem, but looking back on it now, I have come to believe that the stigma of addiction was still being viewed as the individual's problem. Addicts were not ill people to be cured, but bad people.

Purdue Pharma made a great deal of effort to communicate with people of power within the area. Art and the Coalition had put up a web site that included a petition to recall OxyContin. Soon Purdue Pharma's public relations team contacted Coalition members asking to come down to Lee County, talk over the issues with us, and figure out some ways to help. Art quickly gathered some community members whose lives had been affected by OxyContin.

The meeting was held over a meal. Parents of an addicted boy gave a most sensitive story of his family's horrors dealing with the drug. The others present tried to share with the company their professional and personal experiences with having this particularly opioid so easily available. The company representatives continued in their assertion that the availability of the drug was not the problem, addicts were the problem. They offered $100,000 for the Coalition to use as we wanted to work with addicts, if we would take down the OxyContin recall petition from the web site.

The offer did nothing but make the group angry, and things went downhill quickly from there. Greg Stewart, a local pharmacist, left the room. The Purdue Pharma representative pulled from his briefcase an open letter to the public from a doctor who was present in the room. The doctor had already stated, and the letter also stated, two basic tenets: that he was an Appalachian from West Virginia and understood the region; and that OxyContin was not the problem.

Some heated exchanges took place at this point, mine among them, and I also walked out. In the foyer I met Greg Stewart; when I told him I was going to pay for my food, as I didn't want to take anything from Purdue Pharma, he laughed and said he had already done so, for the same reason.

The next day the Purdue Pharma reps met with the sheriff and commonwealth's attorney, among others. The company's offer of $100,000 was being passed around, and apparently Purdue Pharma also gave the sheriff false OxyContin pills to use for sting operations. A few months later, Art was testifying in federal court in Lexington, Kentucky, on behalf of an attorney involved in a suit against Purdue Pharma; there were several lawsuits filed by this time, by lawyers all over the country. Purdue Pharma had a very large legal budget, so most of the time they won. At this trial, company attorneys introduced evidence, a letter from the Lee County sheriff stating that with Purdue Pharma's help the problems with drug abuse had significantly improved. When asked about the letter under cross-examination by Purdue's attorneys, Art testified that he was not aware of any significant improvement.

Meanwhile, parents and victims were starting to communicate with each other through the Internet; sites appeared all across the country sharing information and giving support. Also articles and reports of the significant problem were dominating the media. Greg Wood, a chief health care fraud investigator with the United States Attorney's office, initiated daily e-mail notices that tracked the OxyContin problem nationally, thus helping a host of people all over the country track developments in the OxyContin problem.

Appalachia was forever changed by the availability of this drug: people addicted; families destroyed; grandparents raising grandchildren because the middle generation was in jail, high, or dead. Lee County tried. We tried hard. But our efforts were fragmented, and smaller than they needed to be in the bigger picture.

East Kentucky has been one of the few examples of an area able to work together to develop a community based professional approach to addressing the addiction issues — rather than simply relying on a law enforcement and incarceration approach, as was prevalent throughout the rest of the region. The program UNITE (Unlawful Narcotics Investigations, Treatment and Education) "works to rid communities of illegal drug use through undercover narcotics investigations, coordinating treatment for substance abusers, providing support to families and friends of substance abusers, and educating the public about the dangers of using drugs" (unite.org). UNITE empowers community coalitions to not accept or tolerate the drug culture. In addition to UNITE, Kentucky readily addressed the need for drug courts, and for both short and long term residential treatment programs:

> Drug Court is a shining example of Kentucky's success in specialty courts. Instead of spending time in jail, eligible participants complete a substance abuse program supervised by a judge. Drug Court graduates are more likely to return to productive lives and stay gainfully employed, pay child support and meet other obligations. Today Kentucky has built and are building state

owned and operated treatment facilities throughout the State, and community involvement and education is a significant focus of their approach [http:// courts.ky.gov/courtprograms/drugcourt/Pages/default.aspx].

Although each has developed statewide and local programs, most states in central Appalachia have yet to embrace the challenge of addiction in their population with such practical efforts as drug courts. Most efforts are still grass roots, or handle addiction as a criminal problem, or fall within the purview of the Community Services Board and Mental Health Agencies. During the late 1990s, many different professions, victims and families were talking with each other about the problem and what needed to be done; this faded as the twenty-first century unfolded and each agency began to develop its own take on what addiction was and how it should be tackled. Central Appalachian states could have had a wider influence on other states and federal authorities as the "epicenter," in the same way that northern Maine could have, but for this fragmentation and the very real stigma of being rural, and thus considered undereducated and incapable of self-help. The Virginia Organizing Project; Kentuckians for the Commonwealth; Save Our Cumberland Mountains and other grass roots groups had the intellectual, social and sometimes even the economic capital to be partners in taking on Purdue Pharma — but the agencies seemed mired in the same organizational limit as the government groups. State lines and differences in approach blocked cooperation.

The U.S. Attorney's office out of Roanoke did obtain criminal indictments against three top executives of Purdue Pharma and the company itself. The president, top lawyer, and former chief medical officer of Purdue Frederick, a holding company for Purdue Pharma, each "pleaded guilty to a misdemeanor charge that it had fraudulently claimed to doctors and patients that OxyContin would cause less abuse and addiction than competing short-acting narcotics like Percocet and Vicodin." Purdue was fined more than $600 million. The three executives received 400 hours of community service each, with the judge going on record as regretful that he could not sentence them to jail time (*New York Times* July 21, 2007). Brian Jones, a local organizer for the Virginia Organizing Project, did a great deal to help make the date of the sentencing of the executives a special event for people from all over the country who came to watch the men being sentenced in federal court in Abingdon, Virginia. Judge Jim Jones did a wonderful job of allowing everyone with family members affected by the drug to speak.

While this lawsuit was the first of many for Purdue Pharma, causing the company significant damage over the years, it did little to stem Oxy-

Contin's effects on central Appalachia — or anywhere else in the United States. OxyContin was in the vanguard of a growing, national, prescription opioid problem. By 2013, statistics showed that about 16,000 Americans a year died from prescription opioid overdoses (Meier 2013).

Shortly after the Purdue Frederick executives pled guilty for their actions, Purdue Pharma launched a new marketing campaign, and continues to make a significant profit from the sale of their pain medication. During the years since, several state attorneys general offices investigated Purdue Pharma and brought lawsuits. West Virginia won one of the larger settlements, $10 million, in 2004; use of the funds remains a contested issue in Charleston (*WV Record* 2012). As of 2007, Purdue Pharma has not been allowed to participate in any federal health program for fifteen years, which probably had the biggest impact on the company; that decision was upheld in 2012 in *Friedman et al. v. Sebelius* by United States Court of Appeals for the D.C. Circuit.

What's Working Now

Among others, journalist Barry Meier has written about Purdue Pharma, explaining the results of the company's actions and its impacts on communities, and Purdue Pharma's own bottom line. Meier's 36-page e-book *A World of Hurt: Fixing Pain Medicine's Biggest Mistake* appeared in May 2013. Articles that continue to expose the history of OxyContin and other painkillers, and that investigate links between pharmaceutical representative visits and incentives, and doctors prescribing, continue to shed light on some of the darker sides of an ever-present story.

Kentucky's drug courts work, but even as the program has been modeled by other state, Kentucky's funding is under threat. In 2012, a $25 million budget cut has reduced participants by as much as one-third (alcoholmonitoring.com). Perhaps the most effective ongoing tool in fighting OxyContin locally has turned out to be the Internet. It allowed all kinds of people to immediately communicate happenings all over the country. It specifically allowed people within the region to share their stories. (Don't let the old story about people in rural areas not having computers fool you; we are savvy, literate, and online.) It cost practically nothing for people with limited resources to tell their stories — and to hear from others. And it was a place to share information: what different communities, organizations, families had tried; what worked and what didn't; who had sued whom, with what result; prevailing trends, etc.

Grassroots organizational groups often struggle within themselves to make alliances with stigmatized communities, be those low-income, low-education, or addicted people. State organizations tend to tell rural localities what is going to happen, rather than ask what they need. The inability of state and local organizations to work together, and to work with key stakeholders, hampered what could have become regional alliances working to confront addiction in all its facets. People meant well, but effectiveness would have required overcoming cross-class, cross-educational stereotypes. And that was a win for Big Pharma, a loss for the community.

Conclusion

I still cry when I think about Little Paul — and a multitude of others in our region — lost to prescription drugs. There is hardly a family untouched in the region. No matter how we shout, it seems that the voices of those with money and political clout are easier to hear. Voices without accents. Voices without the rasp of coal dust, or sawdust, in them. Those voices can be heard loud and clear, but ours cannot.

For now. Because those of us who live in rural America — who make the electricity used in almost every house, who hewed the wooden beams that hold up those homes — we are not backing down, going away, or giving up. We are here, and we have a story to tell. Slowly, steadily, case by case, book by book, story by story, we will be heard.

And we will change this story. We must. Our future depends on it.

References

Bourdet, Kelly. 2012. "How Big Pharma Hooked America on Legal Heroin." October, http://motherboard.vice.com/read/how-big-pharma-hooked-america-on-legal-heroin (accessed 21 July 2013).
Karmasek, Jessica. 2012. "Legal Battle over Purdue Pharma Funds Nearing End." *West Virginia Record.* August 10, http://wvrecord.com/news/245990-report-legal-battle-over-purdue-pharma-funds-nearing-end (accessed 13 July 2013).
Meier, Barry. 2007. "3 Executives Spared Prison in OxyContin Case." *The New York Times.* July 21, http://www.nytimes.com/2007/07/21/business/21pharma.html?_r=0 (accessed 13 July 2013).
Meier, Barry. 2013. *A World of Hurt: Fixing Pain Medicine's Biggest Mistake.* Amazon Digital Services. (Accessed 21 May 2013).
Van Zee, Art. 2009. "The Promotion and Marketing of OxyContin: Commercial Triumph, Public Health Tragedy." *American Journal of Public Health* Vol. 99 (February): 2.
Van Zee, Art. 2012. "Cutting Drug Court Budget May Cost Kentucky More in the End." June 7, http://alcoholmonitoring.com/blog/2012/06/cutting-drug-court-budget-may-cost-kentucky-more-in-the-end/#.UelQ420_-00 (accessed 20 July 2013).
Van Zee, Art. 2012. "Ropes and Gray Alert: Government Enforcement." August 1, http://www.ropesgray.com/~/media/Files/alerts/2012/08/ (accessed 20 July 2013).

PART TWO: CULTURALLY APPROPRIATE HEALTHCARE DELIVERY SYSTEMS

Blending Primary Care and Behavioral Health: An Ideal Model for the Diverse Cultures of Appalachia

BOB FRANKO

A case manager who serves people challenged with serious mental illness in northeast Tennessee tells an interesting story about helping a patient. That area of the state is noted for its cascading beauty of the Appalachian Mountain range with its rolling terrain, jutting rock walls and forested peaks. Deep ravines channel dozens of creeks and rivers that flow from the changing elevations of high pastures through dense forests along their journey. However, torrential rains and snow melt-off can almost instantly turn those quiet babbling brooks into swollen powerful rivers that overrun roads, flood valleys and isolate residents for days until the waters subside. Such was the case one day when the case manager received a panicked phone call from a patient. The man was without his medication and roads leading into and out of his mountain hamlet were flooded; there was no telling when the waters would recede for him to get to the pharmacy. He was willing to walk seven miles to where a bridge had washed out to meet the case manager if she could somehow manage a way to get to him.

The case manager knew that a simple hand-off would be impossible. She went to the pharmacy and picked up the medications, a small novelty bucket, and some packing materials. Stopping at home for her fishing gear, she then went to the river's edge. With her patient on the other side, she wrapped the prescription bottle tightly in bubble wrap, secured and waterproofed it with duct tape in the small bucket, tied it to her fishing line, and began trying to cast it as far across and upstream the river as she could get it. It took a few heaves, but she was eventually able to cast the medication across the river to the man who was able to snag the bucket out of the water.

"It's no big deal," the case manager said later. "It's just part of the job."

She still works for Cherokee Health Systems, a safety net provider in east Tennessee. Cherokee Health Systems (CHS) is both a community health center and a community mental health center. It has served the area since 1960 and has grown to 55 clinical locations in 14 Tennessee counties today. Founded as the Mental Health Center of Morristown on the second floor above a bank, CHS began its initial foray into primary care in the late 1970s. A University of Tennessee–educated psychologist, Iowa native Dennis Freeman, was hired as the CEO in 1978 and began an outreach to primary care effort in 1980. Dr. Freeman established some contacts with local primary care providers and began seeing patients in those settings.

The Growing Need for Centralized Services

When asked if they would mind coming to the mental health center for their appointments, very often primary care patients would reply "no way." They were far more comfortable receiving their mental health care in the primary care setting. Stigma was — and remains — a powerful obstacle preventing patients from engaging mental health services, but so was (and is) transportation, cost and access. Thus began a period of "circuit riding" where Dr. Freeman would travel to various sites throughout the week on a regular basis to see patients.

Soon realization dawned that not only was the population of east Tennessee challenged with mental health care access, but with access to health care in general. This was particularly true of patients of CHS, who often had comorbid physical illnesses that exacerbated their mental health issues, and vice versa. The few services available were fragmented and delivered in isolation; providers shared little if any communication. Poverty, unemployment, substance abuse and poor housing compounded the overall health crisis that had formed into a veritable Gordian knot. It was clear to Dr. Freeman that if CHS could centralize and blend primary care and mental health, it would ease some of the bottlenecks that crimped access to care, as well as address the stigma and fragmented care issues.

In the early 1980s, the Clinch Mountain Regional Health Center Corporation was formed as an amalgamation of CHS's services and the Blaine Medical and Dental Board, and shortly thereafter CHS's first primary care clinic was opened in Blaine.

Today, from those roots, CHS provides an integrated primary behavioral health delivery model that addresses the myriad complexities of patients' physical, behavioral and relational issues. It is CHS's belief that the connectivity and interplay between one's physical status and behavioral presentation are so related that the treatment delivery system has to be comprehensive and blended in order to be truly effective and efficient. Often the conditions are so intertwined it is impossible to tease them apart. The questions about where to find skilled behaviorists to work in this model, and payers to support it, have provided plenty of challenges, not only for CHS but for other safety net providers across the country interested in the same approach. Likewise, the prevalence of chronic health diseases, generational poverty, unemployment, substance abuse, lack of health insurance and limited access continue to plague areas of the Appalachian region, prompting care providers to find creative and innovative measures to respond to the incredible demand with precious few resources.

If only the answer were as easy as casting a bucket of medications across a washed out bridge.

Confounding Factors Create Intertwined Diagnoses

One way to appreciate the impact that health disparities has had on the Appalachian region is to concentrate on a specific diagnostic chronic condition. Consider diabetes mellitus, a group of metabolic diseases including Type I diabetes, Type II diabetes and gestational diabetes. Patients experience high blood sugars that may have profound consequences on their overall health status and quality of life, yet in many cases the symptoms and potential further complications (including cardiovascular disease, renal failure, and retinal damage) can be mitigated and controlled through medical and behavioral interventions which support the patient in making lifestyle changes. While it is important to understand the prevalence of this chronic disease on people in the Appalachian region, it is even more important to understand the cultural influences of the region that often impact prevention, diagnosing, treatment and compliance factors. We will consider those factors after gaining more of an understanding of the problem at hand.

A recent study completed by the U.S. Centers for Disease Control and Prevention (CDC) Division of Diabetes Translation published in the *American Journal of Preventative Medicine* identified a diabetes belt located primarily through the southern portion of the United States (Barker et al.,

2011). A map overlay of the counties studied actually depicts two distinct fingers of the belt; one extends through the deep South region including much of the states of Louisiana, Mississippi, Alabama, Georgia and South Carolina. The other portion encompasses much of Tennessee and extends on a path that follows the Appalachian Mountains through much of eastern Kentucky, southwest Virginia, most of West Virginia and a portion of southeast Ohio. In fact, when coupled with obesity, it is established that of the counties identified in the Appalachian swath, 81 percent of them were in the top 40 percent for both conditions (Gregg et al., 2009).

Looking at the prevalence of diabetes alone in Appalachian counties designated as distressed as compared to those non-distressed (or "attainment counties"), another study found that residents of the distressed counties had a 13 percent prevalence rate of diabetes, the attainment counties had a 6 percent rate, versus the national average prevalence rate of 8 percent (Barker et al., 2010). The convergence of diabetes and obesity in these areas is thought to be rooted in the prevailing social and cultural norms, community and environmental influences, socioeconomic status, and hereditary factors (Gregg et al., 2009). These findings certainly support the empirical observations made by many providers and healthcare administrators familiar with the region. Within the population of east Tennessee, CHS providers often comment about the culture and the diet of the patients seen in their clinics. Sweet teas, highly-caffeinated sugary sodas, deep-fried foods and meals cooked using lard and shortening remain as staples of many patients' diets. This is in large measure due to unexamined traditions; lifelong residents of the region were raised on similar diets.

Another factor is the influence of tobacco. A 2006 study found that there was a greater than the national average of tobacco use in Appalachian Ohio, a phenomenon that was found to be replicated across the rest of the Appalachian region (Behringer and Friedell 2006). The study authors describe tobacco as even more of a cultural influence in Appalachia than in other regions around the country because of its deep-seated and historical dependence on tobacco growing and cultivation. They relay that families in the mountainous area often describe tobacco as the "Christmas crop" because the timings of the payments from their crop sales came at that part of the year.

Another strong socioeconomic predictive influence on health disparities in Appalachia is the prevalence of poverty and unemployment. Any healthcare provider can provide anecdotal evidence about the overall poor health of the uninsured population and number studies have found the same. A 2008 project studied the healthcare services utilized by people in southwest Virginia; there the researchers found that there was little difference in the type of healthcare utilized between individuals with private health insurance and those with public insurance. However, they found that those without any insurance at all were eight times as likely to use the emergency room as their primary source of care and were much more likely to delay seeking treatment until their health status reached a critical stage. This is particularly significant when considering that 41 percent of the people in their study were without health insurance, leading the researchers to logically conclude that health insurance is a critical factor in influencing health outcomes (Manton and Thorton 2008).

Even if individuals have insurance, however, there are fewer per capita providers in the region compared to the rest of the country, particularly behavioral and health providers. The Institute for Health Policy Research looked at 618 nonmetropolitan counties in 13 Appalachian states and found that 70 percent of them were designated as a mental health professional shortage area, a ratio higher than non–Appalachian, nonmetropolitan counties within the same states (Hendryx 2008, 179–182). In terms of health services, the U.S. Department of Health and Human Services reports on its website that of the 55 counties in West Virginia, only four are not designated as a Medically Underserved Area or Population (MUA/P). In fact, 91 percent of counties designated as "distressed" in the Appalachia region are designated as Health Professions Shortage Areas, a likely potential factor as to why residents tend to seek care far later in the disease process rather than accessing prevention services prior to onset (Barker et al., 2010).

Stereotypes: The Unspoken Confounding Factor?

Beyond the more easily captured data of disease prevalence, tobacco use and socioeconomic factors, however, still another factor influences the health outcomes of Appalachian residents. It is a more difficult influence to flesh out and measure, but may be among the strongest influences overall: the region's cultural beliefs and norms.

Hollywood, television and literature have created a disparaging caricature of Appalachia and its people. A 2006 study investigating how social and cultural factors influence health in an Appalachian community found that many of those stereotypes are hollow representations of the population and their beliefs. The researchers in particular looked at fundamentalism, isolationism, familism (setting the needs of the family above one's own) and fatalism as characteristics identified with the region, examining how those characteristics influenced choices the population makes in regards to health care. The study participants acknowledged the prevalence of poverty in their region, but rejected the popular notion of widespread extreme poverty that included "someone with no shoes on, living in a shack ... back up in the mountain, up in the hills. No running water. No TV. Probably no refrigerator. With no food.... And we're not like that" (Coyne, Demian-Popescu and Friend 2006). In fact, the study identified positive attributes that residents felt better described their region: friendly, God-fearing, proud, law abiding, hard-working, clannish, and reluctant to share family problems.

Still, there remain pockets of severe poverty as described by various charities and agencies. The Appalachian Poverty Project, a component of the Community Foundation of Carroll County (Maryland), is designed to help get new and gently used appliances to those in need in Appalachia. The organization's website describes the "hollows" across the region as areas deep in the mountains that have been abandoned by the coal industry and resettled by "squatters" who are typically very poor, live in substandard housing, often with illegal electrical hook-ups that resulted in periodic electrocutions.

As it is with any stereotype, it is important to separate fact from fiction and dispel the myths that commonly misrepresent a population or region in regards to a stereotype. Socioeconomic factors are often misconstrued as cultural indicators. For example, recently many states have adopted policies to drug test welfare recipients. Alabama, Florida, Oklahoma, Louisiana, Ohio and Indiana are among those that have contemplated or have introduced bills to mandate the testing based on a belief that welfare recipients use illicit substances at a higher prevalence than others. "Drug testing proponents like to argue that there are large numbers of drug users going on welfare to get money to support their habits," wrote columnist Adam Cohen in *Time Ideas.* "The claim feeds into long-standing stereotypes about the kind of people who go on welfare, but it does not appear to have much basis in fact," he wrote. Cohen cites several studies and the early results of the policy in Florida that indicates that "...as a government policy, drug testing is being oversold" (Cohen 2011).

A policy brief by the National Poverty Center also supports Cohen's argument; an April 2004 brief that states "the authors suggest that policymakers and analysts have likely overstated the contribution of substance dependence to welfare receipt." It further states that poor education, lack of transportation, physical and mental health problems, and other difficulties are more common among welfare recipients than substance abuse and are significant barriers to self-sufficiency (Jayakody et al., 2004). Clearly it is a mistake to stereotype a given population based on socioeconomic indicators. This rings true with the popular misconceptions about people living in Appalachia. Likewise it would be a mistake for physicians, policy-makers and other health professionals to ignore the rich diversity of the population and rely on stereotypes in designing health delivery systems and in improving the health literacy of the region.

A Potential Solution

Lack of access and the health disparities have led to several innovative responses. Cherokee Health Systems has utilized a suite of "tele-services" to reach the underserved. Using high quality videoconferencing equipment, CHS providers can "beam into" remote sites and provide basic health examinations, psychiatry consultations and most recently, pharmacy consultation. One application of this innovative technology has been a partnership between Cherokee Health Systems and the Sevier County, Tennessee, school district. Collaborating on the Student Medical Assistance Response Team (S.M.A.R.T. program), school nurses at 17 elementary and middle schools in the district have access to telemedicine equipment that is securely linked with a CHS provider. A student can be screened, examined, diagnosed, treated and monitored through the system. The state-of-art high tech equipment allows the offsite medical provider to examine the patient's ears, nose, throat, lungs, heart rate and skin in coordination with an onsite nurse. The goal is to provide essential healthcare to underserved children, help them remain healthy and in school, which allows their parents not to miss work. Cherokee Health Systems also uses this technology in providing primary care to patients at one of its remote sites, as well as providing a wide distribution of instant psychiatric consultation system-wide to providers who might otherwise have access to a psychiatrist.

Cherokee Health Systems built its integrated primary behavioral health care delivery system with these health disparities, cultural variations and socioeconomic challenges in mind. Circling back to a patient with diabetes, a common diagnosis in a CHS clinic, one finds the advantages of an integrated system both for the patient and provider alike. A patient with diabetes has a full plate of medical interventions, as well as an array of both physical and behavioral changes to consider. Basic medical interventions include glycemic control and monitoring, weight management, thyroid examination, circulation monitoring, frequent blood tests, medication management, as well as frequent monitoring of vision, dental, kidney and pregnancy issues. The myriad behavioral and lifestyle modifications to consider with the treatment are significant, not the least of which is adherence to a medication regiment, drastic changes to diet and menu planning, the introduction of exercise as a daily routine, and in more severe cases the acknowledgement of new limitations, including driving cautions and the challenges of maintaining one's independent living status. A team-based approach that includes a physician and behaviorist, along with ancillary members that might include diabetes specialists, dieticians, case managers and visiting nurses would be a valuable asset to both the patient and provider alike in the achievement of better outcomes. Expanding beyond the diagnosis of diabetes, imagine the benefits of this approach for patients with anxiety, depression, chronic obstructive pulmonary disease (COPD), post-traumatic stress disorder, insomnia, obesity, cardiac issues, pediatric behavioral issues and those who have a history of somatization.

The basic role of the Behavioral Health Consultant (BHC) in Primary Care at Cherokee Health Systems includes:

- Management of psychosocial aspects of chronic and acute diseases
- Application of behavioral principles to address lifestyle and health risk issues
- Emphasis on prevention and self-help approaches, partnering with patients in a treatment approach that builds resiliency and encourages personal responsibility for health, and
- Consultation and co-management in the treatment of mental disorders and psychosocial issues

Functioning in this population based model, the role of the BHC is adaptable and flexible to the needs of the community and population it serves. At Cherokee Health Systems, the BHC is typically a psychologist level provider who has extensive training in bio-psycho-social interventions, brief therapy, and psychopharmacology. Most are classically trained in psychology, but do not practice traditional mental health therapy in their role as BHCs. As there are no doctoral programs that develop behaviorists to practice in primary care, Cherokee Health Systems has an internship program and tends to "grow its own" crop of behaviorists.

Significant variation comes into play across the communities served in Cherokee Health Systems' 55 clinical locations; some locations serve a very rural population, another may be a pediatrics-only clinic, while another serves a high-volume, richly diverse urban community. However, the basic components of the practice remain intact and flex to the needs of that community. As the BHC considers the best approach with a patient, he must think of the following aspects:

- Symptom severity
- Assessment of the patient's readiness to change

- Psychosocial stressors
- Co-morbid conditions
- Patient preferences
- Cultural beliefs
- Access to resources (transportation, childcare, etc.)
- Health beliefs (i.e., perceptions of self-control, fatalism, etc.)

This makes it an ideal model for the varying populations, cultures and needs of Appalachian residents. Let's explore each of these roles of the BHC in relation to the Appalachia population.

Management of Psychosocial Aspects of Chronic and Acute Diseases

Whether a patient walks into the clinic in acute distress or for a regular checkup to monitor his diabetes or other chronic condition, Cherokee Health Systems believes there is a behavioral component that needs to be considered in that appointment. Behavioral aspects have a direct impact on the quality of life and therapeutic outcomes of a person with a chronic medical condition like diabetes. However, there are a large percentage of patients that present in primary care with physical complaints that have no biological basis, even after an array of expensive and sometimes invasive tests and scans.

A variety of studies have concluded that as much as 70 percent of all healthcare visits, in fact, have primarily a psychosocial basis (Strosahl 1998, 139–166; Fries et al., 1993, 321–325; Shapiro et al., 1985, 1033–1043). More specifically, the ten most common problems presented in primary care are:

- Chest pain
- Fatigue
- Dizziness
- Headache
- Swelling
- Back pain
- Shortness of breath
- Insomnia
- Abdominal pain
- Numbness

While these ten complaints account for 40 percent of all visits, the physician can identify a biological basis for the complaint in only about 15 percent of the visits (Kroenke and Mangelsdorff 1989, 262–266). Among the most common and most frightening for the patient is chest pain and complaints of heart racing, which often have no biological basis. Moderate to severe anxiety is well known to cause elevated respiration and even hyperventilation, symptoms often misidentified as cardiac distress by the patient. Hyperventilation can lead to hypocapnia, or reduced levels of carbon dioxide in the blood, which in turn can cause the chest to tighten, and result in dizziness and breathlessness.

Clearly a patient experiencing these symptoms may become frightened, which has the compounding effect of exacerbating the symptoms. Researchers studying the effects of biofeedback on somaticizing patients have found that an effective intervention for patients presenting with these symptoms may be breathing training. It is believed that as patients learn to control their respirations they can eliminate hypocapnic distress and return their carbon dioxide levels to normal (Nanke and Rief 2004, 133–138). In most cases this will be a far more effective and less invasive intervention for the patient, and more efficient use of the physician's time and overall healthcare resources.

Another frequent complaint is insomnia. Director of Integrated Care, Parinda Khatri, PhD, often describes to visitors a request that many CHS providers hear: almost daily patient requests for the "butterfly pill." A popular sleep medication is heavily advertised on television during prime-time hours. The commercial features a beautiful, gentle butterfly silently gliding over people comfortably sleeping under plush blankets. Yet, while exploring their sleep hygiene habits with the BHC, the patient requesting this pill often describes a diet high in caffeine and sugar, and/or a stressful lifestyle. They often also describe inconsistent sleep patterns or work different shifts.

In these situations the Behavioral Health Clinic and the primary care provider prefer to collaborate on a behavioral approach before considering a pharmacological treatment. The BHC will consult with the patient on several lifestyle modifications including the avoidance of alcohol, caffeine and nicotine in the hours before sleep, as well as avoiding eating heavy foods or consuming lots of fluid before bedtime. The BHC may work with the patient on establishing a more regular bedtime and wake pattern that may include decreased napping, a warm bath before bed, and regular exercise. The primary care provider and BHC may also assess the patient for sleep apnea and counsel him on the use of a CPAP machine if necessary. Helping the patient increase his self-resiliency, the BHC may also request that the patient keep a sleep diary for a period of time, or complete a weekly sleep log. It is important that the BHC recognize the very real experiences of the patient and not discount them as imagined or construed in order to build trust and form a partnership with the patient focused on problem solving. It is also important that this approach be holistic, examining each aspect of the patient's life.

Physicians may also engage the BHC to help treat a variety of other acute care and chronic diseases by focusing on medication adherence, weight management, smoking cessation and cases of high medical utilization by a particular patient. Often high utilizing patients have complaints about poor pain management. Pain management clinics have popped up all over the country, but are particularly abundant in various areas of Appalachia. In 2002 the U.S. Drug Enforcement Agency identified eastern Kentucky among the highest ranking regions in terms of OxyContin abuse. The history of painkiller use in Appalachia may have its roots in the coal industry. The National Drug Intelligence Center reported in its July 2002 *Kentucky Drug Threat Assessment* that coal mine camp doctors would often dispense painkillers to miners who spent hours each day crouched in tight spaces. Self-medication became a way of life for the workers. Having a skilled behaviorist embedded in the team of a health center in areas with a high prevalence of painkiller abuse would be highly advantageous to the patients and clinic alike.

A study completed by the American College of Osteopathic Family Physicians in July 2011 wanted to see if there was a reluctance of Appalachian physicians to prescribe opioids as an effective treatment. In fact what the study found was that more predominant barriers to pain reduction were:

1. Patient reluctance to make lifestyle or behavioral changes
2. Inadequate access to pain specialists
3. Inadequate access to health care because of financial burdens
4. Lack of an objective measurement of pain
5. Physician reluctance to prescribe opioids (Remster and Marx 2011).

It is safe to assume that a skilled behaviorist on staff would be a valuable tool for a physician to help a patient at least contemplate making some lifestyle modifications. After a thorough assessment by the physician, the patient may work with the BHC to explore behavioral practices that can assist the patient better manage his pain. The BHC may teach the patient a number of skills including deep breathing, progressive muscle relaxation and massaging. She may also work with the patient on reframing their perceptions of the pain through journaling and distraction techniques.

Of course the BHC will tailor this approach based on the patient's readiness to change, education and health literacy level and any customs or belief systems that may impact the care. Again, the focus is on a holistic approach not just to primary care, but to lifestyle choices and mental health.

With the prevalence of diabetes, obesity, and issues related to smoking in the Appalachia region, one clearly sees the benefits of the integration of behavioral health in primary care. A frequent question about this practice, though, is about the referral process to the behaviorist. How does the physician introduce the concept to the patient? Isn't there resistance from the patient about seeing a "mental health expert?"

We'll discuss the communication between a physician and a patient — particularly in context of Appalachia — in the section on building resiliency and personal responsibility for health. For now, it is sufficient to point out that in Cherokee Health's history of providing this blended care approach, it has found that patients by-in-large place a great deal of faith in their doctor and if she recommends a particular course of treatment or the involvement of another specialty, patients generally comply. That said, the language the physician uses to introduce the behaviorist is vital. Cherokee Health Systems providers tend not to think of the involvement of the behaviorist in a case as a "referral." Instead it is simply an engagement of a team member, swiftly responsive and choreographed through a "warm handoff."

The physician may identify a situation where a BHC could provide benefit for the patient, for example, to assist with sleep hygiene issues. He may tell the patient that he has a team member who has experience in this area and has a lot of terrific resources that might help him rest better without the use of a potentially addictive sleep agent. The warm handoff is a choreographed brief meeting between the patient, physician and behaviorist usually right in the exam room to get everyone on the same page in terms of the problem and potential solutions. At that point, the physician has "handed off" the patient and leaves the room to attend his next appointment.

Later, the behaviorist will update the physician on her recommendations to the patient, usually through both a brief verbal exchange and through her documentation in the patient's record. The reimbursement for this value-added service is a complicated process that differs from state-to-state based on the policy of payers. Generally most states allow for multiple services on the same day from different providers, but which services are allowable and by what particular discipline tends to have some variance across the states. However, once payers understand the benefits of this cost effective care model, they readily provide reimbursement.

Application of Behavioral Principles to Address Lifestyle and Health Risk Issues

Another of the key roles of a behaviorist in primary care is the application of behavioral interventions to address lifestyle issues and risks to health and wellness. One can easily see the benefits of behavioral support for a person with diabetes, for example. Cherokee Health Systems' core beliefs include that every primary care encounter has a behavioral component, so a primary care office is a virtual incubator for behavioral health involvement in wellness, prevention and treatment. However, it is vital that the practice consider carefully the culture of its patients and any regional variations in beliefs and values that may have either a negative or positive impact on the effectiveness of basic interventions.

Consider tobacco use. We need not tread the well-worn path of the dangers of tobacco, both of the smoking and smokeless variety. How individuals perceive those dangers, however, is widely varied and influenced a great deal by local culture. A recent study in Appalachia examined the influence of tobacco on the region; it found that there is a link between lower socioeconomic status and a higher prevalence of smoking, and since poverty is widespread in Appalachian communities, there is a higher prevalence of smoking than other communities throughout the United States. The study found that the Appalachian region produces 97 percent of the burley tobacco in the United States (Caldwell 2010). Recall tobacco's history in Appalachia as an economic driver, its status as "the Christmas crop." Researchers examining effective anti-tobacco campaigns have long recognized this economic influence and its contribution to the acceptance of tobacco use and why certain strategies common in tobacco education programs outside Appalachia are often ineffective within the region.

It is important to consider both the environmental and cultural influences in the approach when it comes to tobacco awareness in Appalachia. It is a recent trend among states and local governments to enact smoking bans in public places such as restaurants, workplaces, bars and arenas. In Appalachia, neither Alabama, Kentucky, Mississippi, South Carolina nor West Virginia have such laws on the books. Virginia, North Carolina, Georgia and Tennessee have some state bans pertaining to smoking in state offices, restaurants and bars, although with great variation and a number of qualifying clauses.

For example, Georgia only includes in its smoking ban restaurants that allow people under the age of 18 to enter. Tennessee excludes bars altogether, and also prevents local governments from enacting laws tougher than those of the state in relation to smoking bans. The lack of strong state support in the Appalachian region for restricted tobacco use in public places strikes a blow to an effective anti-tobacco campaign according to a study released in the American Journal of Public Health. That study concluded that in the states without a state ban on tobacco use, local ordinances often had a very weak influence.

Said lead author of the study and associate professor of epidemiology at Ohio State University, Amy Ferketich in a May 13, 2010, edition of *Science Daily*: "A lot of people working in tobacco policy suggest that smoking ban efforts have to start in communities before moving to the state level, but we strongly believe that that is not the best model for every state. Based on our findings in these states, with the exception of West Virginia, we recommend that attempts to enact clean indoor air laws must be made on a statewide level to work. Clearly, leaving the effort to the local communities does not result in a large number of strong local indoor air ordinances in these states" (Caldwell 2010).

In other words, if the state does not deem it a priority, why should local governments, and then conversely, why should individuals? Much of Appalachia is "tobacco country," but also "coal country." Miners often use smokeless tobacco while on the job deep underground because they can't "light up" for fear of explosion. A focus group sponsored by the Ohio Department of Health completed by the Voinovich Center for Leadership & Public Affairs in 2004–2005 gathered data on populations dispropor-tionately affected by tobacco use. The report, *Voices of the Appalachian on: Tobacco use, tobacco control, and the effects of tobacco,* cited a focus group participant who offered this observation: "Smokeless tobacco is huge in this area. And it's part of the culture. That's truly just a part of the culture. My grandmother chewed tobacco. And these days you don't hear of women chewing tobacco, but she was from the hills of Kentucky. She chewed tobacco and it's just such a part of our culture.... Everybody does it."

A physician simply telling a patient that he should stop smoking will likely be no more effective in the states of Appalachia than it would be in Michigan or Arizona, but may have the added detriment of leaving the patient feeling as if the doctor has made a judgment on his culture and/or environment. A study examining the use and beliefs of tobacco in Appa-lachia concluded that it is vital that a provider understand the role of tobacco for people in the Appalachians in order to better devise effective strategies to prevent or reduce smoking in this population (Ahijevych et al., 2003, 93–102).

A skilled behaviorist familiar with local customs, culture and belief systems can align themselves with those influences while assessing patients' readiness to change. They might take time to explore a patient's experiences and familial history with tobacco and further explore with the patient the cognitive dissonance between their family's past — and perhaps current — economic dependence on tobacco, and the harm and risk it poses his physical health without judging or condemning. The provider might encourage self-reliance and acknowledge the challenges ahead concerning weak state indoor clean air laws that will cause great temptation for relapse due to the very real physical influence of the smell of smoke and being around others smoking, as well as a fall back to the fatalistic belief of "well, if the state doesn't care, why should I?"

An approach where the behaviorist recognizes the cultural and societal norms of the community and integrates them in their intervention as positive leverage can be quite effective. To do the opposite, to immediately go on the attack of tobacco, risks immediately alienating the patient and would likely lead to unfavorable outcomes. In Appalachian regions, it would not be uncommon to work with a patient who has some perceived positive connection to tobacco through family or personal history. To this day, many Appalachian residents recall with fondness the "Chew Mail Pouch Tobacco" ads painted prominently on the sides of barns throughout Kentucky, Ohio, Pennsylvania, South Carolina, West Virginia and Tennessee.

In fact, even from just an economic standpoint, a wise behaviorist appreciates the uphill battle tobacco prevention efforts face. In 2001 alone, it was reported that the entire tobacco industry spent $11.22 billion promoting cigarettes, and $236 million more to market smokeless tobacco products (Meyer et al., 2008, 67–74). Even though in 1998 some of the major tobacco companies agreed to curtail or stop some of their marketing efforts, by 2012 the U.S. Surgeon General reported that the five largest tobacco companies alone were still spending nearly $10 billion a year on cigarette marketing, a 48 percent increase since 1998 as reported by Michael Felberbaum in an ABCNews.com article on March 8, 2012. An appreciation of all of these factors in the design of treatment interventions for an Appalachian resident will have the most benefit for the patient and provider alike.

Prevention, Self-Help, and Partnering with Patients in a Treatment Approach

Encouraging patient responsibility for one's own health is a key component of Cherokee's approach. Often, a significant role of the behaviorist in a primary care setting is breaking the patient's habit of being a patient. A few high utilizing patients in a practice consume a disproportionate amount of the provider's time and resources. Ask any nurse or receptionist in any doctor's office or community clinic about their "frequent flyers," and they'll rattle off a handful of names of patients who consume inordinate time and resources. While there is little doubt that some of these patients are genuinely ill and need higher levels of care, there is also plenty of anecdotal and statistical evidence that for others their complaints are rooted in non-biological causes (Strosahl 1998, 139–166; Fries et al., 1993, 321–325; Shapiro et al., 1985, 1033–1043).

Behaviorists can play a key role with these patients in developing self-help tools to use instead of continuing to access costly and unnecessary care. While we're certain that this phenomenon holds true throughout Appalachia and across the country, a factor on the far other side of the scale is also true: the vast numbers of patients that are underserved and who avoid medical care all together. There are many reasons as to why patients in general avoid the doctor, be it lack of insurance, unreliable transportation, fear of doctors, or just a lack of providers in a given area. Each of these factors play a role in Appalachia to be sure; however, other factors are just as prevalent and even more difficult to overcome. These include poor health literacy and unique cultural influences that create chasms between providers and potential patients.

Health literacy has evolved from a philosophy to a movement, and now is recognized as a component of a sound practice approach. Still a young and developing practice, health literacy was defined by the U.S. Department of Health and Human Services in its *Healthy People 2010* report as "the degree to which individuals have the capacity to obtain, process, and understand basic health information and services needed to make appropriate health decisions." Under the Patient Protection and Affordable Care Act of 2010, Title V, the definition was slightly expanded to include the term "communicate," as in the degree to which an individual can communicate basic health information and services in order to make health decisions. In 2004 the American Medical Association and its Medical Student Section (MSS) convened a Community Service Committee (CSC) that held its first Health Literacy Month in October 2004. It set out to alert the general medical community on several key facts including:

- 47 percent of adults in the United States read below an 8th grade level
- When statistical adjustments were made for education and other sociodemographic co-variables, literacy level was the strongest correlate of health knowledge and disease management skills

- Health literacy is a better predictor of one's health status than: age, income, employment, ethnicity, or education level
- Studies have shown that low literate patients have poor knowledge and management of their chronic diseases
- Low health literacy negatively impacts patient health

Commonly, vulnerable populations with low health literacy include the elderly, minority and immigrant populations, people defined as low-income, and people with chronic mental and/or physical health conditions. Given the level of poverty alone throughout much of Appalachia, beyond the education and other socioeconomic factors, it is a fair assumption that poor health literacy is a major contributing factor to health care in the region.

Consider the role of poor health literacy in the following example of a recent new patient of Cherokee Health Systems. He told the behaviorist that a couple of years ago he went in for a check-up from his family physician because of a few nagging complaints of heart burn and poor sleep. The man is middle aged, slightly obese, has a history of heart disease in the family and smokes over a pack of cigarettes a day. The physician ordered a lipid panel, a simple blood test that measures total cholesterol, HDL and LDL cholesterol levels and triglyceride levels in the bloodstream; all important risk factors in the development of coronary artery disease. The patient's levels were found to be in the high risk area: His triglycerides were above 600 mg/dL (recommended to be below 200 mg/dL) and his cholesterol numbers were likewise high (or in the case of HDL, low). His blood pressure was also abnormally high. He said he was given some brief counseling by the physician as to what it all meant, saying that "he said I was a good candidate for a heart attack real soon," and that he was given some poorly copied handouts on a low-sodium, low-cholesterol diet and told to start exercising.

On his way home from the appointment he and his wife stopped at a McDonald's for burgers and sweet tea. He said he looked at the handouts and could make little sense of the information as it recommended intakes in terms of milligrams and used terms such as carbohydrates and proteins. He said he felt dumb because he wasn't sure if he was eating any of the foods mentioned on the handouts or not. "Besides," he said, "I thought that if I'm going to go because of a heart attack, I guess that's just the way it is."

Does this case sound familiar? Put into its proper context, one can quickly see the enormous challenges for what would otherwise be a fairly common and simple course to treat. Consider first the patient's environment;

he lives in a distressed Appalachian county that offers few choices for grocery shopping, but has plenty of 24-hour convenience stores, cigarette outlets, liquor stores and some sort of fast food option at almost every intersection. One survey of convenience stores in an Appalachian county found that none of the convenience outlets carried fresh or frozen green or yellow vegetables, low-fat milk or yogurt, or low-fat cheese (Barker et al., 2010). Next, even though the gentleman is a high school graduate, when looking at the handouts he could not translate the information into anything useful; the foods on menus at fast food joints and in the frozen food sections are not listed as carbohydrates or proteins and he had a difficult time conceptualizing metric measurements. Also, the patient is a lifelong Appalachian region resident, a place where residents are characterized as proud, private, wanting to "take care of their own" (Behringer and Friedell 2006). He didn't want to burden anyone else with his problems, nor did the encounter with the physician heighten his level of trust of the medical community; in fact, it just caused him more fear. Reading the gentleman's statement about a looming heart attack just being "the way it is," one sees marks of a fatalistic attitude.

Clearly, a lack of health literacy is a compounding factor contributing to the increasingly alarming risk factors this particular patient has; in any of the environmental factors described above, even some incremental increase in the level of health literacy could have a positive impact on his choices. Perhaps he would better associate the foods he would normally eat with those described on the handouts the physician gave him; perhaps he would make better choices while dining out. Perhaps he would recognize his own role in the state of his overall health instead of casting it to the winds of fate.

Situations like these are a perfect fit for a behaviorist. It is an opportunity to form a connection with the patient based on the behaviorist's understanding of the patient's environment, culture and values, and helping him gain insight to his role in his health. At Cherokee Health Systems, the gentleman met with a behaviorist who spent some time to educate him on what some better choices would be in terms of menu planning and food selections when shopping or eating out using real-world examples since she was very familiar with the area. The next time it might be to spend some time reviewing the lipid panel results and teach him what the indicators mean and offer one or two things he could start to do to change them. It is a teaching moment to increase the person's health literacy to help him achieve better health outcomes.

Mention was made of the patient's trust of the medical community. A study focused on a community in southern West Virginia and found that there was a fair amount of distrust of physicians. The participants noted that going to a doctor or emergency room was regarded as a "last resort" fearing that their family problems will become public, or that they will be given medications that will cause addiction (Coyne, Demian-Popescu and Friend 2006). Further numerous studies have found a general distrust of foreign-born physicians. Cultural differences between foreign-born physicians were cited as barriers to trust, as well a lack of cultural competence on the provider's part, and that some health care professionals belittle patients for the speech patterns and idioms (Coyne, Demian-Popescu and Friend 2006; Barker et al., 2010). Again, this is another perfect fit for a behaviorist to intervene not only for the patient, but also in team meetings to help educate the provider staff on local customs and beliefs.

Consultation and Co-Management in Treating Mental Disorders and Psychosocial Issues

We've well established the impact of behavioral health issues in primary care, particularly those that are incident to a medical condition. However, another prominent role for a behaviorist in primary care is to help intervene when there is an emerging mental health issue during an appointment. Consider a fairly common situation at one of Cherokee Health Systems' clinics.

A parent scheduled a "sick visit" for her teenage son who complained of an ear ache. Upon arrival the patient was asked to complete a standard screening form that contained a variety of questions including those related to depression. As the patient was about to be taken to an exam room to begin his appointment his questionnaire was scored and found that he provided some red flag scores in the depression realm. The physician was alerted to this before entering the room and during the course of his examination of the patient's ears — he was, indeed found to have an ear infection — he explored the depression issue with the patient. After some initial resistance, the teen admitted to having rather significant depressive thoughts including passive thoughts of harming himself.

The physician said that he had a teammate who might be helpful to him and excused himself to go get the BHC. They chatted briefly about the situation on their way back to the exam room, and after introductions conducted a brief co-interview with the patient, and then as the BHC took over the discussion, the physician quietly exited and moved on to his next appointment. He and the BHC communicated a short time later about the outcome. It was decided that the teen would benefit from — and agreed to — returning in a week to check in with the BHC after picking up a few tools to cope with his depression and better assess where he is at that point. The BHC was comfortable that the teen was not actively suicidal or in danger of harming himself after the initial discussion, but was prepared to offer whatever level of support he needed. The teen eventually began regularly checking in with a school counselor and still asks to say hello to BHC whenever he returns for routine medical care.

Without the screening mechanisms to detect an underlying and potentially emergent mental health disorder, the physician would have been blind to the problem. Further, without adequate training in mental health treatment, or without the referral resources and integrated approach to care, the depression would likely have gone undetected. If by chance it did emerge in the primary care visit, without the built-in resources available to this provider the likely course of care would have been a referral to a local mental health provider (a majority of which are not followed up on), or even a prescription for an antidepressant. The challenge for providers in Appalachia for issues such as this is compounded by additional stigma to mental health services, as well as few culturally sensitive trained providers to work effectively with people from the region.

Providers in the region benefit from an appreciation of the unique cultural values of Appalachian people, including: religion, independence, self-reliance and pride, neighborliness, familism, personalism, humility and modesty, love of place, patriotism, sense of beauty, and sense of humor (Jones 1994). A few of those values particularly important for providers to recognize include the importance of modesty and humility, personalism, and some degree of fatalism or "what will be, will be" attitude as we saw in our adult patient discussed earlier.

In his book *Appalachian Values*, Loyal Jones, retired director of the Appalachian Center at Berea College in Berea, Kentucky, states that people from Appalachia (or "mountain people" as he refers to them) are "levelers," meaning they tend to believe they are as good as anybody else, but not necessarily better than anybody else; they place tremendous value in modesty and humility. They tend not to be boastful or put on airs (Jones 1994).

This is useful knowledge for counselors, as Heather Ambrose, PhD, assistant professor of counseling and human services at Lindsey Wilson College in Columbia, Kentucky, and Roger D. Hicks, M.Ed., Magoffin County Protection and Permanency, Salyersville, Kentucky, explain in their paper "Culturally Appropriate Counseling and Human Services in Appalachia: The Need and How to Address It": "If a non–Appalachian counselor approaches an Appalachian client as if he/she is an expert and therefore better than the client, the client will automatically become distrustful of the counselor."

Reflect back to the interaction between the physician and the teen with depression; the physician was not judgmental or prescriptive. He acknowledged the issue and introduced a teammate who is "might be helpful to him." A kinship, or "leveling" was created through his choice of words; instead of introducing the BHC as a trained psychologist trained to treat people with depression (which may have been interpreted as "she's better than you"), he created a team concept with the patient included.

Personalism, according to Jones, is another trait unique to the Appalachian culture. It is the general desire for an Appalachian to relate well with others. Jones said that since it is important for people from Appalachia to get along with others, he or she may sometimes agree with another person when in fact they do not. Certainly this could have an impact on the counseling relationship. If the patient does not trust the provider, he may agree to setting up next appointments and completing any number of tasks in the meantime, but in reality has no intention of following through with any of it. Jones said these behaviors are often interpreted by outsiders as Appalachians not being reliable. Ambrose and Hicks state that it is imperative that a counselor be aware of this tendency and be even more diligent to build a collaborative, trusting relationship with the patient. Again, reflecting back on our teen patient it is clear that the BHC built a level of trust with the patient as he agreed to the tasks assigned and the followed up as requested.

There is some debate in the literature as to the degree of fatalism that exists throughout Appalachia. We saw a degree of it in our adult patient, but researchers tend to have different opinions as to its impact on Appalachian residents' decisions to access health care (Beringer and Friedell 2006; Jones 2006). Religion and faith are strong values in the Appalachian culture, and there is evidence that people who live in the region place equal value in their faith and directions from health professionals when making their health care decisions (Beringer and Friedell 2006). Others believe that fatalism isn't necessarily the "what will be, will be" attitude in the context of Appalachia; rather it is that because of the wealth of social problems that exist in the region, residents there simply have a general feeling of hopelessness.

Counselors can reframe this feeling by utilizing some of the positive values attributed to Appalachians including self-reliance. It might be necessary to use a more confrontational or challenging approach to "rally" the patient by pointing out the discrepancies in his thinking (Ambrose and Hicks 2006). Think again of our adult patient and one of the techniques employed by the BHC; the plan to sit down with the patient and through an educational approach to increase health literacy, the idea to build the patient's self-reliance by going over the lipid profile results and teaching him areas where he had direct control. It is important to not de-value the patient's faith in the process — to recognize his external locus of control through his faith — but to identify and bolster the opportunities the patient has to exercise more control himself.

These are just a few of the factors that a well-trained, culturally sensitive provider understands in their approach to working with the unique population of Appalachia. Reflecting back to our initial discussion of patients with diabetes, it should by now be clear the number of "touch points" or intervention opportunities an integrated practice has for patients diagnosed with diabetes. Understanding the actual treatment implications can help better define preventative measures throughout the practice starting even in pediatrics by focusing more heavily on diet and exercise for at-risk children.

Making the Case for Integrated Care in Appalachia

An approach to health care that integrates primary care and behavioral health is an ideal practice for safety net providers around the country, but particularly in Appalachia. A team approach that includes an interactive multidisciplinary panel of medical practitioners, psychologists, psychiatrists, nurses, dieticians, counselors, case managers and pharmacists — among others — is the only way to effectively address the myriad physical and psychosocial issues of a population. Rampant poverty, inadequate housing, near epidemic levels of chronic disease, substance abuse, health disparities, lack of access to health care and a dwindling number of new general practitioners entering the system are some of the major challenges and obstacles faced in Appalachian communities.

At Cherokee Health Systems we often say that our patients come to us fully assembled, so it is vital that their health care system be likewise fully assembled to meet their needs. It might be as accurate to say that the obstacles to overall health listed above are as functionally fully assembled. They are as interconnected as are the relationship between a person's mental, behavioral and physical conditions. Poverty is as connected to inadequate housing as it is to depression and so on. We are all familiar with the cycle of poverty. An integrated approach to care recognizes and responds to these interconnected issues. No primary care visit is without a behavioral component, whether it is through lifestyle and health risk issues, or through prevention and the building of health literacy and advocating for patient self-reliance.

The demand for services of the safety net population shows no signs of decreasing, and in fact, all signs point to increased demand. Finding new, innovative approaches to meet that demand is our ongoing challenge. It is also our duty to never let the manifest demand obstruct the unpresented need.

References

Ahijevych, K., Kuun, P., Christman, S., Wood, T., Browning, K., and Wewers, M.E. 2003. "Beliefs about Tobacco among Appalachia Current and Former Users." *Applied Nursing Research* 16: 93–102.

Ambrose, Heather J., and Hicks, Roger D. 2006. "Culturally Appropriate Counseling and Human Services in Appalachia: The Need and How to Address It." *American Counseling Association VISTAS Online,* http://counselingoutfitters.com/Ambrose.htm (accessed 9 March 2012).

American Medical Association. Medical Student Section, Community Service homepage, http://www.ama-assn.org/ama/pub/about-ama/our-people/member-groups-sections/medical-student-secton/community-service/health-literacy.page# (accessed 6 February 2012).

Appalachian Poverty Project. The Appalachian Poverty Project homepage, http://www.app-pov-proj.org (accessed 5 February 2012).

Barker, Lawrence E., Crespo, Richard, Gerzoff, Robert B., Denham, Sharon, Shrewsberry, Molly, and Cornelius-Averhart, Darrlyn. 2010. "Residence in a Distressed County in Appalachia as a Risk Factor for Diabetes, Behavioral Risk Factor Surveillance System, 2006–2007." *Preventing Chronic Disease* 7, no. 5 (September), http://www.cdc.gov/pcd/issues /2010/sep/09_0203.htm (accessed 8 March 2012).

Barker, Lawrence E., Kirtland, Karen A., Gregg, Edward W., Geiss, Linda S., Thompson, Theodore J. 2011. "Geographic Distribution of Diagnosed Diabetes in the United States." *American Journal of Preventative Medicine* 40, no. 4.

Behringer, Bruce, and Gilbert H. Friedell. 2006. "Appalachia: Where Place Matters in Health." *Preventing Chronic Disease* 3, no. 4 (October), http://www.cdc.gov/pcd/issues/2006/oct/06_0067.htm (accessed 30 January 2012).

Caldwell, Emily. 2010. "Community Approach to Smoking Bans not Effective in Appalachia, Study Finds." *Science Daily* (March 6), http://www.sciencedaily.com/releases/2010/05/100513162746.htm (accessed 6 March 2010).

Cohen, Adam. 2011. "Drug Testing the Poor: Bad Policy, Even Worse Law." *Time Ideas* (August 29), http://ideas.time.com/2011/08/29/drug-testing-the-poor-bad-policy-even-worse-law/ (accessed 6 February 2012).

Coyne, Cathy A., Demian-Popescu, Cristina, and Friend, Dana. 2006. "Social and Cultural Factors Influencing Health in Southern West Virginia: A Qualitative Study." *Preventing Chronic Disease* 3, no. 4 (October), http://www.cdc.gov/pcd/issues/2006/oct/06_0030.htm (accessed 30 January 2012).

Fries, James F., Koop, C. Everett, Beadle, Carson, Cooper, Paul, England, Mary Jane, Greaves, Roger F., Sokolov, Jacque J., and Wright, Daniel. 2012. "Reducing Health Care Costs by Reducing the Need and Demand for Medical Services." *New England Journal of Medicine* 329: 321–25.

Glassman, Penny. 2011. National Network of Libraries of Medicine, Health Literacy homepage, http://nnlm.gov/outreach/consumer/hlthlit.html (accessed 6 February 2012).

Gregg, E.W., Kirtland, K.A., Caldwell, B.L., Rios Burrows, N., Barker, L.E., Thompson,

T.J., Geiss, L., and Pan, L. 2009. "Estimated County-level Prevalence of Diabetes and Obesity, United States, 2007." *Morbidity and Mortality Weekly Report* 58, no. 45 (20 November), http://www.cdc.gov/mmwr/preview/mmwrhtml/mm5845a2.htm (accessed 30 January 2012).

Hendryx, M. 2008. "Mental Health Professional Shortage Areas in Rural Appalachia." *Journal of Rural Health* 24, no. 2: 179–182.

Jayakody, Rukmailie, Danziger, Sheldon, Seefeldt, Kristin, and Pollack, Harold. 2004. "Substance Abuse and Welfare Reform." *The University of Michigan-Gerald R. Ford School of Public Policy-National Poverty Center-National Policy Brief*, no. 2 (April), http://npc.umich.edu/publications/policy_briefs/brief02/ (accessed 6 February 2012).

Jones, Loyal. 1994. *Appalachian values*. Ashland, KY: The Jesse Stuart Foundation.

Kroenke, K., and Mangelsdorff, A.D. 1989. "Common Symptoms in Ambulatory Care: Incidence, Evaluation, Therapy and Outcome." *American Journal of Medicine* 86: 262–266.

Manton, Marian R., and Thorton, Gwendolyn B. 2008. "Healthcare Services Used by Appalachians in Southwest Virginia." *Sociation Today* 6, no. 2 (Fall), http://ncsociology.org/sociationtoday/v62/health.htm (accessed 30 January 2012).

Meyer, Michael G., Torborg, Mary A., Denham, Sharon A., Mande, Mary J. 2008. "Cultural Perspectives Concerning Adolescent Use of Tobacco and Alcohol in the Appalachian Mountain Region." *Journal of Rural Health* 24, no. 1 (June 4): 67–74.

Nanke, Alexandra, and Rief, Winfried. 2004. "Biofeedback in Somatoform Disorders and Related Syndromes." *Current Opinion in Psychiatry* 17, no. 2 (March): 133–138.

Ohio Department of Health. 2006. Voices of the Appalachian on: Tobacco Use, Tobacco Control, and the Effects of Tobacco. Voinovich Center for Leadership & Public Affairs, http://ohiocctca.org/Ohiocctca/Documents/Population%20Reports/Appalachian%20Report.pdf (accessed 5 March 2012).

Remster, Erin N., and Marx, Tracy L.. 2011. "Barriers to Managing Chronic Pain: Perspectives of Appalachian Providers." *Osteopathic Family Physician* 3, no. 4 (July): 141–148, http://www.osteopathicfamilyphysician.org/article/S1877-537X(10)00114-0/abstract (accessed 15 February 2012).

Shapiro, Sam, Skinner, Elizabeth A., Kramer, Morton, Steinwachs, Donald M., Regier, Darrel A., and Fein, Rashi. 1985. "Measuring Need for Mental Health Services in a General Population." *Medical Care* 23: 1033–1043.

Strosahl, Kirk. 1998. "Integrated Primary Care Behavioral Health Services: The Primary Mental Health Care Paradigm." In *Integrative Primary Care: The Future of Medical and Mental Health Collaboration*. Alexander Blount. New York: Norton.

U.S. Department of Health and Human Services. 2010. *Healthy People 2010*. Washington, D.C.

U.S. Department of Justice. 2002. *Kentucky Drug Threat Assessment*. National Drug Intelligence Center. Washington, D.C.

U.S. Department of Justice. *OxyContinTM*. Drug Enforcement Administration, http: www.justice.gov/dea/concern/oxycontin.pdf (accessed 30 January 2012).

Telehealth in Appalachia

Steve North, MD

"Mary" is a seventh grader who lives in the town of Spruce Pine, North Carolina, halfway between Asheville and Boone. Four years ago Mary was diagnosed with cystic fibrosis following a series of difficult-to-treat lung infections. Mary began seeing pediatric pulmonologists at the Cystic Fibrosis Center at the University of North Carolina (UNC CF). When she is healthy, Mary sees her doctor in Chapel Hill, North Carolina — a four-hour drive from Spruce Pine — every three months. Unfortunately, during the 2012-13 school year Mary had an increased number of lung infections and was seen in Chapel Hill three times during the first four months of 2013. Mary missed more than twenty days of school for doctors' appointments in Chapel Hill, although she fortunately was never hospitalized (M. McGee and McGee 2013).

Mary's mom "Ann" is a registered nurse. While Ann recognizes that the care at UNC is excellent, when asked about her experiences she quickly identifies the significant costs for Mary to be seen in Chapel Hill so frequently. These costs include Ann taking days off from work, staying in a hotel room, at least a tank of gas per trip, and the cost of food. Ann estimates that between expenses and lost income each visit costs their family $500 in out of pocket expenses (M. McGee and McGee 2013).

Ironically Mary's school, Harris Middle School in Spruce Pine, is part of the MY Health-e-Schools (MYHeS) school-based telemedicine program and since October 2011 has had a telemedicine unit capable of connecting to UNC from the school nurse's office (McCall 2013). According to Ann, when she asked why Mary could not be seen via telehealth for regular follow-up visits, she was told that the UNC CF Center has questioned the ability of the local hospital to replicate the pulmonary function tests that are performed at every visit to UNC.

Telehealth in Saltville, Virginia

Approximately 100 miles away from Mary's school, and across the state line, patients with cystic fibrosis are seen by their specialists at the University of Virginia in Charlottesville (UVa) via telemedicine from the Saltville Medical Center, part of the Southwest Virginia Health Systems, Inc. Federally Qualified Health Center. Since the Saltville program's inception in December 2012, Sally Pennings, a family nurse practitioner there, states that there has been a high level of acceptance of telehealth cystic fibrosis care by both the patients and providers (Pennings and North 2013). Using an integrated telehealth system that combines interactive videoconferencing, a stethoscope that connects via Bluetooth to the computer, a video otoscope (in lay terms, an ear microscope) and a fiber-optic laryngoscope that streams real time images, Pennings facilitates the clinical visit at the Saltville site. Working with the physicians at UVa, she uses the equipment to thoroughly examine the patient, including the nasal cavities for recurrent polyps. Combined with locally performed pulmonary function tests and labs, patients in Saltville are able to be seen for both acute and regular visits that reduce — but do not entirely eliminate — the need to make the 500 mile round trip to Charlottesville.

Pennings has led the development of the Saltville, Virginia, telehealth program since its inception in 2001, and feels that the distance to specialists at UVa and other tertiary care centers is not only a barrier to patients receiving the best care possible, but also contributes to patients "surrendering to their illnesses." She sees benefits for both the patients and the providers in offering telehealth services. Personally she reports feeling more connected to the patient and their disease process because she is "more involved in their care," and believes that she develops a greater understanding of the specialists' concerns when she participates in the visit.

As Mary's situation illustrated, merely having access to telehealth technology does not guarantee that a patient can connect to the needed provider or services. Throughout Appalachia the penetrance and utilization of telehealth technologies is highly variable. A few communities are extremely well connected. The entire state of Virginia is a model of telehealth delivery. However, many states and communities in Appalachia are struggling to determine how to use telehealth to improve access to healthcare and overall health outcomes. Using three telehealth programs in Mitchell County, North Carolina as starting points, we will explore the current and potential impact of telehealth on rural Appalachia and the barriers to its increased acceptance and implementation.

Mitchell County, North Carolina's Telehealth Programs

Currently three programs exist in Mitchell County, each operated by a different entity and targeting a different and fairly specific health issue. While Mitchell County is beginning to feel the impact of telehealth on direct patient care, often neither the providers nor the patients are clear about how to best use the available programs. The oldest, a telepsychiatry program located at the Bakersville Community Medical Clinic (BCMC) has been operating since 2010. Using videoconferencing and a dedicated T1 line, patients in Bakersville connect with a psychiatrist approximate 60 miles away in Asheville. T1 lines are digital communications lines that carry a maximum of 1.544 megabytes per second (mbps). Often, as used at BCMC, a T1 line is employed for dedicated point-to-point videoconferencing as a means of preserving bandwidth and ensuring privacy. The MYHeS telemedicine program, launched in October 2011, currently provides school-based telemedicine services at ten schools in Mitchell and Yancey counties. In January 2012, Blue Ridge Regional Hospital launched telestroke program in its emergency connecting patients with stroke-like symptoms to stroke neurologists at Mission Hospital in Asheville. The development and growth of these programs serve as models to explore the current and potential impact of telehealth on Appalachian communities and the current, potential and perceived barriers to this technology reaching its full potential.

Mitchell County is like many other rural Appalachian counties in that it struggles with high rates of chronic unemployment, substance abuse, and limited access to health services. In Mitchell County the aging population has growing health care needs that are increasingly difficult to meet in a rural area with limited health infrastructure. Additionally, the total population of the county has decreased steadily over the past ten years, resulting in fewer working-class young families (*State and County Quick-Facts* 2013). These three factors have a direct and synergistic effect on the region's economic stability and educational resources in addition to the health care system. In the past 15 years Mitchell County has lost nearly two-thirds of its manufacturing jobs due to corporate decisions to outsource furniture and textile production. This has resulted in an average unemployment rate of 13 percent and a higher than average percentage of the county's citizens being uninsured or publicly insured than the state population as a whole. Combined with the difficulty in finding primary care providers that most rural communities in Appalachia often face, Mitchell County is a Health Resources and Services Administration (HRSA) designated primary care Health Provider Shortage Area (*Find Shortage Areas* 2012).

Defining the Technology

Although the words "telemedicine" and "telehealth" are frequently used in discussions of improving healthcare in rural communities, patients and providers in these communities are rarely able to define what this technology entails. "Telehealth" and "telemedicine" are often used interchangeably as their definitions have evolved. However, the American Telemedicine Association defines them as distinctly different from each other:

> Telemedicine is the use of medical information exchanged from one site to another via electronic communications to improve a patient's clinical health status. Telemedicine includes a growing variety of applications and services using two-way video, e-mail, smart phones, wireless tools and other forms of telecommunications technology [*What Is Telemedicine?* 2013].

In contrast, HRSA defines Telehealth as

> the use of electronic information and telecommunications technologies to support long-distance clinical health care, patient and professional health-related education, public health and health administration. Technologies include videoconferencing, the internet [sic], store-and-forward imaging, streaming media, and terrestrial and wireless communications [HRSA: Telehealth 2013].

Both of these definitions are quite formal and do not help to describe the variety of programs that have been implemented in Appalachia, across the United States and in other countries. Telehealth services can range from: a scale in the home of a patient with congestive heart failure, that scale connected to a centralized nursing office; to a rural emergency department having a robot that is operated by a neurologist at a tertiary care center, the robot being used to evaluate a patient having symptoms of acute stroke. This essay will use the HRSA definition of telehealth to describe all programs.

The language of telehealth can be somewhat confusing at times but understanding it is critical because licensure and reimbursement requirements vary from state to state. Not using the correct terminology may result in not being reimbursed. In telehealth, an image of a bicycle wheel has been historically used to describe a network with the provider at the hub and the patients at the spokes. As telehealth networks have become more complex, this image is no longer applicable; the site where the patient is located is referred to as the originating site, while the site where the

provider is located is called the distant site. There are three ways that telehealth services are classified based upon the level of provider-patient interaction and the timing of this interaction: the store and forward telehealth;
interactive telehealth; and remote monitoring.

Store and forward telehealth involves capturing medical data that is
sent electronically to a healthcare provider who reviews the information
at a convenient time. Examples of this include images of a skin rash, microscope images of a surgical specimen, or radiology films. The store and forward method does not require the simultaneous presence of both the patient
and provider at the same time and is generally employed in the medical
specialties of dermatology, pathology, and radiology. Of the three, tele-
radiology is the most frequently employed; digital images on a shared network might be reviewed by radiologists who specialize in a specific image
type, or by a "nighthawk" radiologist literally on the other side of the globe
who provides a preliminary interpretation of emergency room CT scans
to the emergency department physician. While it is possible to use store
and forward telehealth for acute issues by sending a brief history and an
image of— for example — swollen tonsils to a remote provider, public and
private insurers rarely reimburse for this method.

Interactive telemedicine allows a patient to be seen by a remote provider who can ask questions, perform a physical examination with the
assistance of a variety of peripherals and a telehealth presenter, and engage
the patient in the development of a treatment plan. Interactive telemedicine
can occur in a variety of settings: a patient's home through the *Health
Insurance Portability and Accountability Act* (HIPAA) compliant web-based
video software; an ambulance with a paramedic relaying images, EKGs
and other clinical information to an emergency room physician; between
two healthcare settings where an outpatient is being seen for a follow-up
visit; or, in an inpatient setting where an entire intensive care unit is monitored by nurses and physicians located at another facility, possibly in
another state. Interactive telemedicine typically requires the greatest level
of technology and bandwidth and is the most common form to be reimbursed for acute patient care.

Remote monitoring is most often used in a patient's home to look
for changes in a patient's vital signs to anticipate or predict changes in his
health. A simple example is a patient with congestive heart failure whose
scale is connected to a home health agency via a plain old telephone system
(nicknamed a POTS). Daily weights are sent electronically to the agency,
and if the weight changes beyond defined parameters, the computer algo-
rithm alerts a nurse of significant weight. The nurse then calls the patient
and provides instructions on how to treat the condition, potentially pre-

venting an emergency room visit. A more advanced example of home monitoring is an integrated system where a patient's medication box compliance, daily vital signs, and responses to a daily symptom checklist are monitored by a remote nurse. The nurse uses interactive videoconferencing to provide medication reminders, clinical education, and evaluation of changes in the patient's condition. Remote monitoring is one of the fastest-growing areas of telehealth, although high speed Internet is often required in the patient's home for this complex technology to be successfully implemented. Reimbursement for home telemonitoring is state- and insurance-company dependent. However as the evidence of its effectiveness at preventing emergency room visits and hospital admissions grows, more states are moving towards insurance reimbursement for home telemonitoring.

The telehealth presenter is an essential part of the care team. The telehealth presenter is located at the originating site and conducts the visit by operating the equipment, checking vital signs, and sometimes participating in the clinical exam. In the MYHeS program at Mary's school, the school nurse serves as the telehealth presenter, as Pennings does for the Saltville Medical Clinic's cystic fibrosis clinic. The medical provider, located at the distant site, works with the telehealth presenter to examine the patient and provide comprehensive care. Qualifications for a telehealth presenter can range from a twenty-hour training course that covers basic operation of the machine and confidentiality issues, to being a nurse practitioner. Even though they are actively involved in the exam, telehealth presenters typically cannot bill independently for their services; this restriction can present a barrier to comprehensive telehealth care.

A Brief History of Telehealth

Telehealth in the United States has been developing since the 1950s, when the University of Nebraska used television connections to provide mental health services to rural communities in the state. The first large-scale telehealth project in the United States involved collaboration between the National Aeronautics and Space Administration (NASA), the Papago Indians (now known as the Tohono O'odham Indian Nation), the Indian Health Service, and the Lockheed Missile and Space Company. The STARPHAC (Space Technology Applied to Rural Papago Advanced Health Care) (Freiburger, Holcomb, and Piper 2007) program was started in 1973 as an attempt to provide remote evaluation of patients at a reservation village by physicians at the Indian health service hospital located approximately

50 kilometers away. In addition these patients could be seen at the major referral center, the Indian Health Service Hospital in Phoenix, Arizona. The service relied on two-way video, audio, and data communications using microwave, VHS radio and telephone connections to transmit both real-time and store and forward information. The project was active from 1973 until 1977.

The first use of telemedicine in Appalachia appears to have been in December 1974 with the launch of the Ohio Valley Medical Microwave Television System ("Microwave Brings Telemedicine to Appalachia" 1976). Described as an "ultra-modern system" this project was developed to address the decreasing number of physicians practicing in Ohio's Appalachian Region Health Demonstration Area. The Appalachian Region Health Demonstration Area encompassed seven counties in southeastern Ohio as well as the cities of Athens and Gallipolis. The program installed full-service television studios in the O'Bleness Memorial Hospital, the Mental Health Care Center in Athens, and the Holzer Medical Center in Gallipolis. These facilities were connected to the Ohio State University Hospital in Columbus via a dedicated microwave television system, and were used to provide patient consultations and medical education. In addition to the television delivery, a component of the microwave system could transmit heart and lung sounds from moving ambulances in the seven county area to the nearest hospital for early evaluation and treatment of pulmonary problems. This was as important as it was useful at a time when volunteers who were not paramedics operated most ambulance services. This network operated until 1980, when it was replaced by newer technologies.

Funding for many early telehealth programs in Appalachia came from the Appalachian Regional Commission's (ARC) Telecommunications Regional Initiative (1995–1998) and subsequently the ARC's Information Age Appalachian Program. The goal of the later program was to "stimulate economic growth and improve the overall standard of living in the region by funding projects that focus on building access to infrastructure infusing telecommunications technology and business sector and cultivating the skills and knowledge of the region citizens to use the technology effectively"(Kleiner et al., 2003). An analysis of the ARC's funding suggests that of the seventy telecommunications projects funded by the Appalachian regional commission from 1994–2000, seventeen of the programs had a goal of improving "consumers' access to quality healthcare" (Kleiner et al., 2003). In further evaluation of these 17 programs, six reported having more success than they expected in improving the access to healthcare, while two were less successful than anticipated.

Telepsychiatry

"Cathy" is 21 and has been seen via telepsychiatry at the Bakersville Community Medical Clinic in North Carolina for the past three years. She started these televisits following an emergency hospitalization precipitated by severe depression, racing thoughts, auditory hallucinations and an inability to sleep. She had been discharged from a state hospital on very strong antipsychotic medications that caused her to gain a lot of weight and feel groggy and unfocused. Through a series of telepsychiatry appointments, it became clear to the psychiatrist that she was suffering from bipolar affective disorder rather than a psychotic disorder. Under the direction of the psychiatrist she was able to be tapered off her antipsychotic and antidepressant medications, which exacerbated the symptoms of her bipolar affective disorder. This case is one example where, without the ability to link with a psychiatrist, the patient would likely have remained on the antipsychotic medications for a much longer period of time before being correctly diagnosed and treated.

Since June 2010, Bakersville Community Medical Center has been providing telepsychiatry services in cooperation with the Pisgah Institute, a private psychiatry practice located in Asheville. One half day per week a consulting psychiatrist is available through a videoconferencing system to provide both direct patient care and consultations to primary care providers. This project was initiated by the Western Highlands Network, one of the Local Management Entities (LMEs) developed by the state of North Carolina to develop and regulate mental health services for uninsured and publicly insured clients. Since its inception the telepsychiatry program has seen more than 250 unique patients.

Tim Evans, the licensed clinical social worker who coordinates the Bakersville program, feels that the majority of these patients would not have received the needed level of psychiatric care without the telepsychiatry program in place. When asked about patient acceptance of the program (which was the first telehealth program in Mitchell County or any of the adjacent counties) Evans said, "Many patients are initially hesitant about participating in the program, feeling that it will be strange to talk to a television screen. Almost all patients are willing to try one time. I believe that every patient has come back after the first appointment with no further hesitation. There have been several patients who have wanted to see the psychiatrist in person for the first visit and were willing to travel to Asheville to do that. All of them have transferred their care to the telepsychiatry program after that first visit. Each patient who has participated has reported high levels of satisfaction" (Evans and North 2013).

In addition to community based settings, telepsychiatry has been found to have clear benefits for nursing home residents. A multistate pilot program in rural nursing homes analyzed 278 telepsychiatry encounters for 106 unique patients and found that using telepsychiatry saved 843 hours of travel time and a had a potential savings of more than $500 per visit when transportation costs and nurse time for either the patient or the physician were calculated (Rabinowitz et al., 2010). Cost savings to the overall health care system is one of the largest drivers of the implementation of telehealth technologies.

School-Based Telemedicine Needs

"Mrs. Jones, Tommy has an earache and you need to come pick him up to go to the doctor." For all parents, this phone call can completely change the course of their day. Leaving work to drive to the school, hoping to get an appointment at the doctor's office, and then sitting in the waiting room for the last work-in appointment of the day is stressful for parent and child. Especially in rural communities that suffer from lengthy travel times to limited provider locations accessed by curvy roads, kids like Tommy often end up in the emergency room at 7 p.m.

If Tommy lived in Mitchell or Yancey counties in western North Carolina, he could have been seen at school through the MY Health-e-Schools (MYHeS) school-based telemedicine program. The MYHeS program, like all school-based health programs, obtains consent and a medical history from a student's parents at the beginning of the school year. Then, when a student needs to be seen the parent, a teacher, or the student can contact the school-based health center and schedule a visit. In Tommy's situation, using secure videoconferencing equipment combined with peripherals including an otoscope and a stethoscope, he could be examined and his illness diagnosed by a medical provider. The provider could then call the parent and let them know if Tommy needed to go home, prescribe any necessary medications electronically, send a copy of the encounter to Tommy's medical home, and arrange for necessary follow-up. Being seen through MYHeS would allow Tommy to get the care he needs sooner, decrease the stress on his family, and potentially prevent an unnecessary absence.

Accessing comprehensive health services is a great challenge for children and adolescents in rural areas of North Carolina and the United States. *The Well-Being of Children in Rural Areas* (DHHS 2011) illustrates that rural youth in the United States have higher rates of obesity, asthma, untreated depression, dental disease and type II diabetes compared to their urban peers. In addition, rural children are more likely to have public health insurance (SCHIP or Medicaid), live in a HPSA community, and face greater geographic barriers to receiving health care.

For students at approximately 340 rural schools nationwide, school-based health centers (SBHCs) play a critical role in improving access to comprehensive health care to school-age children and adolescents by providing medical care, mental health and counseling services, family outreach, health education, and collaborative chronic illness management.

Multiple studies have demonstrated the value of school-based health centers on improving access to preventive health care and decreasing emergency room use (Guo et al., 2005; Key, Washington, and Hulsey 2002; Allison et al., 2007). They can also improve the utilization of mental health services (Juszczak, Melinkovich, and Kaplan 2003) and decrease health care expenditures. In addition, the quality of adolescent preventive health care provided at SBHCs has been shown to be equal to that of traditional primary care sites and more likely to include counseling about sexual health and screening for sexually transmitted infections (Klein et al., 2007).

Strong evidence exists that the use of an SBHC also improves academic outcomes for the students who use it. In a study of high-risk adolescents, those who used their SBHCs had a meaningfully significant increase in their attendance and grade point averages (Walker et al., 2010). Users of SBHCs have been shown to be less likely to drop out of high school in studies of both the general population (Kerns et al., 2011) and expectant young mothers (Barnet et al., 2004). This clear connection between health and academic outcomes demonstrates how school-based health centers meet the Institute for Healthcare Improvement's Triple Aim of improving the care of individual students, improving the overall health of the student population, and reducing the per capita costs of health care delivery (Berwick, Nolan, and Whittington 2008).

School-based telemedicine programs are relatively new in the scope of school-based health care, with the first programs being less than ten years old. Growing evidence supports that this delivery mechanism improves access to care and decreases stresses on families (McConnochie et al., 2010). In an early study, the use of school-based telemedicine prevented a parent or guardian from missing an average of 3.4 hours of work time and saved approximately $101 to $224 for each visit (Young and Ireson 2003). The University of Rochester's Health-e-Access program is the most studied school-based telemedicine program in the United States and has demonstrated improved health outcomes and health care utilization. Evaluation of the Health-e-Access program found significant cost savings through the use of school-based telemedicine. If the program prevented 0.5 emergency department visits per child who used the program annually, then the cost of the program would be covered (McConnochie et al., 2007). Additionally, the Health-e-Access program demonstrated that 85 percent of acute visits to primary care pediatrics could be completed through telemedicine (McConnochie, Conners, Brayer, Goepp, Herendeen, Wood, Thomas, Ahn, and Roghmann 2006b) and that the frequency of disagreement on diagnosis between providers remained the same for telemedicine visits and in-person visits (McConnochie, Conners, Brayer, Goepp, Herendeen, Wood, Thomas, Ahn, and Roghmann 2006a). The combined benefits of school-based health services and school-based telemedicine programs must be investigated as a method for reaching rural and low-income children.

MY Health-e-Schools currently improves access to primary care, behavioral health and nutrition services for 4000 students at fourteen schools in Mitchell and Yancey counties in the Appalachian Mountains of western North Carolina. Both counties are designated as primary care and dental Health Professional Shortage Areas.

Unfortunately, financial sustainability is an ongoing challenge for smaller and rural SBHCs due to fewer potential patients and therefore limited income compared to expenses. Currently, SBHCs provide care at less than 2 percent of the rural public schools in our country. Still, school-based telemedicine has the potential to leverage economies of scale to provide evidence-based comprehensive health care to rural youth across our country.

School-based telemedicine programs in the United States tend to be affiliated with a medical school, a large tertiary care center, or a large Federally Qualified Health Center. MY Health-e-Schools is unique in that it is a community-based effort to solve a local issue. While there are multiple benefits to launching a school-based telemedicine program in conjunction with a large organization, there are more rural communities that need improved access to health care than regional health systems, medical schools, and FQHCs prepared to develop these partnerships. The MYHeS model of telemedicine being developed and promoted by the Center for Rural Health Innovation has the potential to help school-based telemedicine grow in communities throughout Appalachia.

Telestroke Care in Rural North Carolina

Cotton, a mason in his mid–60s, presented to the Celo Health Center in November 2010 for a regular checkup. Located in southern Yancey

County, North Carolina, the Celo Health Center is approximately 10 miles from the nearest post office and 20 miles from the Blue Ridge Regional Hospital in Spruce Pine, North Carolina. During the appointment with his physician Dr. Philip Mitchell, he developed some word finding difficulty and a slight facial tic. Mitchell quickly sent him via ambulance to Blue Ridge Regional Hospital. One week earlier Blue Ridge Regional Hospital had officially launched its telestroke program, connecting its emergency department to Mission Hospital, the nearest Primary Stroke Center, sixty miles away in Asheville. Within 47 minutes of Cotton arriving at the hospital, he had undergone a CT scan of his head that was interpreted by a neuroradiologist, been evaluated via telemedicine by a stroke-certified neurologist at Mission Hospital, and received streptokinase. Eighteen months after the onset of the stroke system symptoms, Cotton returned to teaching masonry at the local community college and the regional prison, and felt that he was doing quite well (Mitchell 2013).

Stroke programs across the country focus on the sixty-minute "door to needle" window in which a "clot-busting," or thrombolytic, drug like streptokinase can be administered. Before this medication is administered it is critical that the physician treating the symptoms know what type of stroke the patient is having. There are two types of strokes requiring very different treatment. A hemorrhagic stroke occurs when a blood vessel ruptures and blood enters the surrounding brain tissue. In contrast an ischemic stroke occurs when a blood clot blocks a blood vessel in the brain and causes that part of the brain to die due to a lack of oxygen. Thrombolytic drugs like streptokinase can only be used in ischemic strokes; when they are used within three hours of the onset of stroke-like symptoms, a patient may have an almost complete recovery. Giving a patient with a hemorrhagic stroke a thrombolytic drug can worsen the active bleeding and significantly symptoms. With a telestroke program in place, patients who present to an emergency department with telestroke services can have the same likelihood of receiving thrombolytic therapy as those presenting to a Primary Stroke Center (Demaerschalk et al., 2011).

When a patient presents to the emergency department with stroke-like symptoms, it is the beginning of the critical "Golden Hour" for stroke care. The "Golden Hour" is a national standard for rapid assessment and treatment of a thromboembolic stroke. Within the first ten minutes the patient must be seen by a physician to assess the time of onset and the severity of the stroke. In the first 15 minutes an institution's stroke team must be mobilized (either in person or via telehealth). Within 25 minutes the patient must be in the CT scanner to image the brain and differentiate between an ischemic and a hemorrhagic stroke. Within 45 minutes the patient must be evaluated by a neurologist, the CT scan interpreted, and a clinical decision made as to whether or not thrombolytic therapy is appropriate.

When a regional medical system wants to begin a telehealth program, telestroke care is often their entry point (Fanale and Demaerschalk 2012). One of the reasons for this being a convenient entry point is that multiple for-profit companies exist that provide various levels of plug-and-play telestroke care for hospital systems. One example is the system used by Mission Hospitals and their affiliated regional hospitals. This system employs a telehealth robot operated by a neurologist at the distant site to examine the patient. The distant site and the originating site are connected using a secure proprietary network that is maintained and continually tested by the company that owns the robot. This decreases the need for personnel in the originating emergency department to serve as presenters, allowing them to care for other patients. Mission Hospitals contracts with a private company for the robots at the outlying hospitals and the secure network thereby alleviating some of the technology infrastructure stress on outlying hospitals.

A physician at the Celo Health Center since 1997, Mitchell is also a physician in the Blue Ridge Regional Hospital (BRRH) emergency department. He recognizes that without the telestroke services, Cotton's outcome may have been quite different, due to the distance to Mission Hospital and the potential for worsening condition in an ambulance as opposed to an emergency center department. He believes that the tele-stroke system is beneficial to patients by improving access to quality acute stroke care. However he also recognizes that, while patients may know about the tele-stroke system at BRRH, they often wait too long to present to the emergency department after the onset of stroke-like symptoms and therefore cannot be treated with streptokinase. He believes that the presence of local earlier intervention provides an opportunity for the hospital to increase its community education at the signs and symptoms of stroke and the benefits of early treatment.

Inpatient telehealth services are gaining a great deal of attention throughout the country. These services allow critically ill patients to remain in their communities while their local physicians work with consulting specialists to manage the patient or the patient is managed almost exclusively by providers at another institution. While this is very appealing, an attempt to develop such a program at BRRH has met initial resistance from providers at the major regional hospital due to the lack of critically ill patients. This presents a challenge for small rural hospitals. Larger hospitals are not interested in developing critical care telehealth services because the patients at the rural hospital are not sick enough to justify the time and expense of establishing a telehealth program. Therefore the patients that need a higher level of care are transferred to the tertiary care center. However, until the hospital can offer critical care telehealth services, it is not possible to keep the very sick patients at a small hospital develop the resources needed to care for them. Continuing to send critically ill patients to large tertiary care centers puts strain on patients' families who cannot be present to provide emotional support. Additionally, due to the loss in hospital reimbursement that often accompanies the transfer of a patient, there are not the resources for rural hospitals to train the staff and develop the hospital infrastructure necessary to care for the sickest patients.

Successful Telehealth Outreach Examples

Many strong telehealth programs serve the Appalachia region, including the University of Kentucky, the University of Pittsburgh Medical Center, and multiple regional hospitals. Virginia has one of the strongest statewide telehealth networks, led by programs at the University of Virginia and Virginia Commonwealth University connecting 238 unique originating sites to multiple distant sites. These networks have taken a significant amount of time and energy to develop over the past fifteen years, according to David Cattell-Gordon, head of the University of Virginia's Office of Telemedicine. The Virginia Department of Medical Assistance and the Virginia Tobacco Commission have provided critical support through reimbursement for pilot programs and the expansion of broadband networks into rural Appalachia. In 2010, legislative support for telehealth in the state of Virginia resulted in passage of Senate Bill No. 675 requiring insurers to provide equal reimbursement for telehealth and in-person medical care further strengthening the growth of telehealth networks (Wampler 2010).

Cattell-Gordon believes that one of the greatest challenges in the development of telehealth programs is people underestimating the time it takes. In his experience, multiple factors at both of the community-based originating site and at the large academic center's distant site slow the implementation. Rarely is technology or connectivity the greatest barrier to new program development; instead it is administrative issues, professional politics and legal issues. Each new relationship requires time to develop, build and maintain.

Developing regional and statewide programs similar to those in Virginia is critical to the further growth and long-term success of telehealth programs in North Carolina. Despite having some of the strongest academic medical centers in the country, and the University of North Carolina at Chapel Hill and Duke University, and East Carolina University's School of Medicine being an early leader in telehealth applications historically, there has been little collaboration between these organizations. In 2012 the North Carolina Healthcare Information and Communications Alliance (NCHICA) and in March 2013 launched the Telehealth Resources Center of North Carolina (Anderson 2013). Focused on improving payment sources, sharing business models, defining technical standards and advocating for legislative action, this organization will be critical in advancing telehealth in North Carolina.

Across the state of North Carolina the use of telehealth technology to provide primary care visits or subspecialty consultations is quite limited despite multiple large health systems engaging in some form of telehealth. In contrast, throughout southwestern Virginia outpatient telehealth for subspecialty care has been successfully operating since 2001. Cancer services is one example.

Dr. Sue Cantrell is the director of the Lenowisco Health District, comprised of Lee, Scott and Wise counties and the City of Norton in southwestern Virginia. During the first three months of her job (begun in 2000) she met many women throughout this rural Appalachian area dying from preventable cervical cancer. A combination of no local providers who treated early cervical disease, limited patient understanding of the progression of cervical disease to cancer, and the patients' lack of money or transportation needed to see a gynecologist contributed to this epidemic (Cantrell 2013). As a solution she developed a telegynecology clinic at the local health department, connecting women with early cervical changes to a gynecologist at the University of Virginia in Charlottesville. A video colposcope operated by an experienced family nurse practitioner transmitted images of a patient's cervix to a gynecologist, who could then direct the nurse practitioner to take biopsies for further evaluation, and/or to freeze certain areas to prevent further spread of the disease.

The program was highly successful and led to decreases in the number of cases of advanced cervical disease presenting to the health department clinics. Cantrell soon developed other telehealth networks, including comprehensive care for chronic hepatitis C; endocrinology subspecialty clinics; diabetes education; telepsychiatry; and teledermatology.

Cantrell cautions that the largest successes for both patients and programs seem to occur when the patients are most comfortable with the skills of the trained telehealth facilitator. She believes that the best facilitators are not only skilled at operating the equipment, but also know the community and the local resources. Being able to make a strong connection with the patients improves patient comfort levels with the technology, and also increases the likelihood that patients will return for follow-up visits.

Reimbursement initially was a large barrier to the sustainability of the Lenowisco programs, but in 2010 Virginia passed SB 675 (*Virginia's Legislative Information System* 2013). This mandated parity in reimbursement for interactive telehealth services by all health insurance providers. The passage of this law has led to increased sustainability for existing telehealth programs across the state, as well as expansion, and helped Virginia become a national model for integrated telehealth systems.

Home Health in North Carolina

Due to the region's increasingly aging population, Mitchell County's several home health agencies have begun to explore different types of telemonitoring, but none have launched a full-scale telehealth program yet. An example of a home monitoring program using advanced telehealth equipment is one that uses two-way audiovisual monitors and equipment to measure blood pressure, pulse, temperature, blood glucose and weight in a patient's home. In addition to transmitting vital signs, patients use a touch-screen monitor to respond to daily questions about their specific health condition. Once this information has been collected, if necessary, the home care nurse is able to talk to the patient via videoconference and determine the best treatment for the patient's symptoms.

It is difficult to identify any advanced home monitoring programs in the Appalachian region that have substantial data to support their use. One of the limiting factors may be that broadband connectivity varies throughout Appalachia. This may rapidly change in the near future as the ability to access high-speed internet in Mitchell County, and other rural Appalachian regions, should change drastically due to the federally funded Broadband Initiatives Program (BIP) grant (*NC Broadband* 2013). As part of the American Recovery and Reinvestment Act of 2009, this "last mile" broadband program will allow every home access to 100 mbps broadband. A key question that many Appalachian communities are facing is how to best position themselves to take advantage of this new technology.

Funding

Most telehealth programs have faced significant funding challenges during the course of their development. These programs have high start-up costs directly related to technology and Internet connectivity, while many states lack comprehensive reimbursement mechanisms. Each of the telehealth programs in Mitchell County employed a different mechanism for financing their startup and continued operation of their programs. The Blue Ridge Regional Hospital's telestroke program is funded through the larger Mission Health System as part of the system's operational costs. Though the actual reimbursement for a telestroke visit in the emergency department may not equal the cost of providing the service, the combination of reimbursement received for the overall stroke care and the cost savings seen through early, local treatment offset the cost of the equipment. The Bakersville Community Medical Clinic established the telepsychiatry program in partnership with the Western Highlands Local Management Entity, the quasi-public regional mental health management program. This government agency purchased the telehealth equipment and helps offset the program's ongoing expenses of seeing uninsured patients. The greatest expense has been the T-1 line used to connect the videoconferencing unit to a central bridge for linking to the psychiatrist. The cost of the T1 line is subsidized by the Universal Service Administrative Company's (USAC) Rural Health Fund. This program is funded through the Universal Service fee assessed on every telephone bill and reimburses rural health care providers for the difference in the cost of telecommunications between rates in an urban area and rates in a rural area.

The MY Health-e-Schools program has had the greatest diversity of funding for both equipment and operational expenses. The equipment funding was leveraged over time using sequential grants. An initial $40,000 grant from a local community foundation was matched with funding from the Appalachian Regional Commission to total $120,000 for the first three school sites and the network infrastructure. This funding was then matched with the United States Department of Agriculture's Rural Utilities Service's Distance Learning and Telemedicine Grant to allow the network to expand to an additional seven schools. In addition, the MY Health-e-Schools program has received grants from the Health Services and Resources Administration's School-Based Health Center Capital Grants program to purchase additional telehealth units. Operational funding for the program is currently being received from the Kate B. Reynolds Charitable Trust and two grants from the state of North Carolina focused on improving access to primary care for safety net patients.

All three of these programs submit bills to insurance companies and have received payment for standard E&M codes. Also, an additional "technology fee" or "site fee" is reimbursed to telehealth networks by some insurance companies. North Carolina currently does not have any insurance companies reimbursing for remote monitoring telehealth, limiting its implementation and spread.

Utilization

Utilization of telemedicine services at times does not meet the expectations of the providers who have created the networks. As Cantrell said, "one of the somewhat unanticipated barriers was that even with locally available telemedicine equipment, people were reluctant to go from one county to the next to receive care because finding transportation to the originating sites continued to be a major issue."

Both the MY Health-e-Schools network and the telepsychiatry program at the Bakersville Community Medical Clinic have had difficulty with protecting a rate of utilization and then achieving this rate once it is established. During 2012 approximately 34 percent of patients scheduled to see the psychiatrist via videoconferencing did not keep their appointment. Without the clinical services of the psychiatrist being underwritten by the Western Highlands LME, this project would not have been financially sustainable due to this high no-show rate. Tim Evans, a licensed clinical social worker, shared that while stigma often surrounds seeing a psychiatrist he also believes that the initial thought of seeing a doctor through a television set is a barrier for many patients in this community.

Amanda Martin is the executive director of the Center for Rural Health Innovation located in Bakersville, North Carolina, the parent organization of the MY Health-e-Schools. She shared additional insight into why the MYHeS network is not reaching its goal of "seeing 50 percent of the students at each school two times during the school year." While the program was intended to be fully operational at the start of the 2012-2013 year, the new telemedicine carts were not delivered until early October and the equipment at two of the schools did not work until February 2013. Additionally, MY HeS encountered the same challenges of finding a full time provider that the traditional bricks and mortar clinics in the community face. A full-time provider was not available until January 2013. Since hiring a full time provider and improving the reliability of the technology, use of the telemedicine program, along with parents', students' and teachers' perceptions of the program, have improved significantly.

Barriers

The complexity of licensure for telehealth providers between states and credentialing at multiple medical facilities is currently seen as one of the greatest barriers to implementation. Telehealth providers, whether they are radiologists or cardiologists, need to both be licensed to practice medicine in the state and credentialed to practice at the hospital where the originating site is located. State licensure and hospital credentialing processes are arduous tasks for any physician regardless of their specialty. A specialist planning to see patients at multiple institutions via a telemedicine network this process could become a logistical nightmare. The issues of licensure reciprocity and shared credentialing is being actively addressed by both state and national telehealth advocacy groups in an attempt to ease the expansion of telehealth programs.

As mentioned previously, the state-by-state variation in insurance reimbursement for telehealth services is also preventing the expansion of networks across state lines. One of the South Central Virginia FQHC clinics, Twin City Medical Center is located in Bristol, Virginia and patients from both Virginia and Tennessee are seen there. Patients who have insurance through Tennessee Medicaid are not able to use the extensive services offered at this site because Tennessee Medicaid only reimburses for live video telemedicine for "crisis related services." (*Telehealth Policy* 2013) This example clearly illustrates that the laws governing telemedicine reimbursement limit patients' access to existing programs.

Despite the clear need for telestroke services in rural communities, the barriers to its adoption and further implementation tend to be related to organizational technology development and policy setting (Silva et al., 2012). Additionally the common barriers of government regulation and certification providers and also financing of the telestroke equipment can be a barrier for rural hospitals. Mitchell identified education of the community about the signs and symptoms of stroke as critical in increasing the number of patients who was seen within three hours of the onset of symptoms. A novel program in rural Virginia found that two groups of elderly men who received stroke education at a local community center through either telehealth or in-person had an equal increase in stroke related knowledge (Schweickert et al., 2011). This study shows the potential for telehealth to provide stroke education and other disease specific health education at non-clinical facilities. Providing health education for patients in a variety of settings has the potential to increase their knowledge of both specific disease processes and the resources available to treat the disease.

Placing telehealth equipment in ambulances is a concept that has been deployed in multiple areas in the United States and is being explored in rural Appalachia. Telemedicine-equipped ambulances providing stroke care while in route to the hospital reported disruption of the audio and visual signal in 18 of 30 evaluation scenarios (Liman et al., 2012). These tests were performed in Berlin, Germany, a large metropolitan area with a robust cellular communications network, so it is concerning that even in this built environment, the ambulances were not able to maintain connections necessary to be an effective means of improving care. Considering the implementation of similar mobile evaluation systems in mountainous terrain could be prohibitive. In Mitchell County, two national cell phone companies provide coverage, yet there are many spots throughout the county where there is no cell phone signal. Until a company invests in extending their coverage, cellular communications will not be an option for transmitting information from a moving ambulance. With decreasing population in rural Appalachia, the financial incentive for any for-profit entity to invest more in telecommunications infrastructure does not exist. This is a situation repeated throughout rural communities in United States.

Potential

Amanda Martin, executive director of the Center for Rural Health Innovation, has said:

> There are extremes in our community — poor, illiterate, desperately dependent people who need access to the care that can be provided at school because they cannot, and will not, get it anywhere else. And then there are the educated, employed, yet isolated, families who need services and can get them — but have to make hard choices between working full week at an hourly job or taking off to drive long distances to the doctor. Or maybe it is about getting the best care that is usually only accessible in urban areas, even though they choose to live out in the mountains. Whether it is time or gas money or something else, there are difficult choices being made every day by Appalachian families who want to live in these communities, but risk compromising their health and access to healthcare in order to do it. I see telehealth as an ideal means to increase access to healthcare for all members of our community.

Telehealth is experiencing tremendous growth across the country and its growth is beginning to be seen in Appalachia. The ability to take clinical data collected in almost any setting and have it transmitted to a healthcare provider has great potential to change the way healthcare is delivered in this region. Multiple factors exist that may encourage the hospitals and outpatient providers to embrace telehealth as a means of improving patient outcomes.

Changing health care reimbursement mechanisms now focus on the quality of that care provided to patients as a component for reimbursement. Over time rate health economists and health care leaders believe that this concept, known as pay for performance, will be directly tied to the overall level a physician or healthcare entity receives for the care they provide. A physician whose patients with diabetes have well controlled blood sugars may receive a higher rate of reimbursement for the care she provides than one whose patients have poorer control. In the inpatient setting, Medicare is applying increased focus to preventable hospital readmissions within 30 days of a patient being discharged. As part of the Affordable Care Act, Medicare is able to withhold reimbursement for the subsequent hospital stay when a patient is readmitted for the same diagnosis within 30 days of discharge (*Readmissions Reduction Program* 2013). The diagnoses that are being targeted include heart attacks, congestive heart failure, and pneumonia.

In both of these scenarios telehealth technologies exist that will help healthcare providers receive longitudinal information that will help manage patients more closely. Telehealth options that allow daily home monitoring and transmission of blood sugars, respiratory function, and weight currently exist and have been proven to can assist providers in preventing readmissions and improving patient outcomes. In addition, to use a virtual inpatient consultation with the remote cardiologist pulmonologist prior to discharge may help the patient avoid complications three weeks after discharge. As technology costs fall and reimbursement systems change more hospitals and office practices will be embracing this technology.

The expansion of broadband in rural communities was previously discussed. As broadband access expands, rural communities will continue to become more technologically savvy and will expect more interactive and internet-based solutions to medical issues. Encountering grandparents who Skype or watch streaming movies is not uncommon in any community, and as the baby boomer generation ages and demands more access to healthcare, the expansion of telehealth technology will continue to grow. Dependent upon physician comfort levels and market-based forces, the potential exists for critical access hospitals to be staffed entirely by nurse practitioners with all specialty and subspecialty care delivered via telemedicine. While this concept is currently quite disturbing to many physicians and patients, as the need for primary care and specialty care services grows throughout Appalachia, new cost-efficient ways of connecting patients to the limited number of primary care and specialist physicians will need to be implemented.

The Big Concern

Telehealth is an emerging technology with tremendous potential to impact both the access to healthcare and the long-term health outcomes of a historically underserved population. The cost of telehealth, especially when considering real-time solutions involving electronic stethoscopes, high-resolution video cameras and otoscopes, ophthalmoscopes, is quite expensive and therefore it is difficult for a small medical office to purchase the necessary equipment. As large hospital systems fund the use of tele-health as a means of expanding their regional market share, the potential exists for a single medical office exists to telehealth units placed by multiple competing healthcare organizations. This possible duplication of services and expensive equipment does not fit well with the current goals of reducing waste in healthcare. However, without some level of competition for patients by specialists, the patients will lose the option to choose which providers they see. And sharing equipment seems an unlikely option for competitors for market share.

One alternative to the placement of multiple telehealth units in the same community is to have a single community or FQHC owned telehealth center where connections can be made to a major institution elsewhere, particularly teaching hospitals. To accomplish this it is necessary to re-examine the federal funding of telehealth network development. Instead of large entities being sponsored to extend their webs, the federal government should use regional funding sources like the Appalachian Regional Commission to focus on sponsoring small rural sites with excellent connectivity. Expanding the network from the originating site to the distant sites will allow truly improved access for all citizens while at the same time keeping the overhead cost relatively low. This will also allow other organizations to connect with the community telehealth center and provide services without needing large upfront capital investment, thus maintaining patient's choice of specialty and subspecialty providers.

Telehealth penetrance in Appalachia is currently at a point where developing community telehealth centers is possible and critical to insuring that our community members have choice in the providers that they see. By allowing patients to stay in their own communities the revenue generated from laboratory, radiology and other ancillary services will also remain in the local community and may lead to further job growth in the health professions. Outside of job growth in the health professions there exists the potential for stronger local communities. Business growth outside of the medical is often tied to the availability of high quality, accessible health care. Additionally, expanding the scope of health care services available in a rural community through the use of broadband connectivity has the potential to serve as a model for growth in other business and educational sectors. Growth in jobs and increased connectivity to health care specialists are two pieces of the complex puzzle that will allow rural communities like

Spruce Pine, North Carolina to continue to survive and reduce the burden of disease that Mary and other patients experience on a daily basis.

References

Allison, Mandy A., Crane, Lori A., Beaty, Brenda L., Davidson, Arthur J., Melinkovich, Paul, and Kempe, Allison. 2007. "School-Based Health Centers: Improving Access and Quality of Care for Low-Income Adolescents." *Pediatrics* 120, 4 (October): E887–E894. doi:10.1542/peds.2006-2314.

Anderson, Holt. 2013. "Strengthening Telehealth Programs in North Carolina." Presentation at Health and Telehealth World in Boston, MA, July 25.

Barnet, B., Arroyo, C., Devoe, M. and Duggan, A.K. 2004. "Reduced School Dropout Rates Among Adolescent Mothers Receiving School-Based Prenatal Care." *Archives of Pediatrics & Adolescent Medicine* 158, 3 (March): 262–268. doi:10.1001/archpedi.158.3.262.

Berwick, D.M., Nolan, T.W., and Whittington, J. 2008. "The Triple Aim: Care, Health, and Cost." *Health Affairs* 27, 3 (May 1): 759–769. doi:10.1377/hlthaff.27.3.759.

Cantrell, Eleanor Sue. 2013. Letter. Norton, VA.

Demaerschalk, Bart, Miley, Madeline, Kiernan, Terri-Ellen, Bobrow, Bentley, Corday, Doreen, Wellik, Kay, Aguilar, Maria, et al. 2011. "Stroke Telemedicine." *Mayo Clinic Proceedings* 84, 1 (September 11): 53–64. doi:10.4065/84.1.53.

DHHS, U.S. 2011. "The Health and Well-Being of Children in Rural Areas." Rockville, MD: US Department of Health and Human Services.

Evans, Timothy, and North, Steve. 2013. Letter. "Tim Evans." Bakersville, NC.

Fanale, Christopher, and Demaerschalk, Bart. 2012. "Telestroke Network Business Model Strategies." *Journal of Stroke and Cerebrovascular Diseases* (August 10): 1–5. doi:10.1016/j.jstrokecerebrovasdis.2012.06.013.

Find Shortage Areas. 2012. Health Resources and Services Administration, http://hpsafind.hrsa.gov/HPSASearch.aspx (accessed 22 January 2012).

Freiburger, Gary, Holcomb, Mary, and Piper, Dave. 2007. "The STARPAHC Collection: Part of an Archive of the History of Telemedicine." *Journal of Telemedicine and Telecare* 13, 5 (August 3): 221–223.

Guo, J.J., Jang, R., Keller, K.N., McCracken, A.L., Pan, W., and Cluxton, R.J. 2005. "Impact of School-Based Health Centers on Children with Asthma." *Journal of Adolescent Health* 37, 4 (October): 266–274. doi:10.1016/j.jadohealth.2004.09.006.

HRSA: Telehealth. 2013. Health Resources and Services Administration, http://www.hrsa.gov/ruralhealth/about/telehealth/ (accessed 7 May 2013).

Juszczak, L., Melinkovich, P., and Kaplan, D. 2003. "Use of Health and Mental Health Services by Adolescents Across Multiple Delivery Sites." *Journal of Adolescent Health* 32, 6, S (June): 108–118. doi:10.1016/S1054-139X(03)00073-9.

Kerns, Suzanne E.U., Pullmann. Michael D., Walker, Sarah Cusworth, Lyon, Aaron R., Cosgrove, T.J., and Bruns, Eric J. 2011. "Adolescent Use of School-Based Health Centers and High School Dropout." *Archives of Pediatrics & Adolescent Medicine* 165, 7 (April): 617–623. doi:10.1001/archpediatrics.2011.10.

Key, J.D., Washington, E.C., and Hulsey, T.C. 2002. "Reduced Emergency Department Utilization Associated with School-Based Clinic Enrollment." *Journal of Adolescent Health* 30, 4 (April): 273–278. doi:10.1016/S1054-139X(01)00390-1.

Klein, Jonathan D., Handwerker, Lisa, Sesselberg, Tracy S., Sutter, Erika, Flanagan, Erinn, and Gawronski, Beth. 2007. "Measuring Quality of Adolescent Preventive Services of Health Plan Enrollees and School-Based Health Center Users." *Journal of Adolescent Health* 41, 2 (August): 153–160. doi:10.1016/j.jadohealth.2007.03.012.

Kleiner, Brian, Silverstein, Gary, Long, Kelly, Raue, Kimberley, Setzer, Carl, and Wells, John. 2003. "Evaluation of the Appalachian Regional Commission's Telecommunications Projects: 1994–2000." Report prepared for the Appalachian Regional Commission.

Liman, T.G., Winter, B., Waldschmidt, C., Zerbe, N., Hufnagl, P., Audebert, H.J., and

Endres, M. 2012. "Telestroke Ambulances in Prehospital Stroke Management: Concept and Pilot Feasibility Study." *Stroke* 43, 8 (July 23): 2086–2090. doi:10.1161/STROKE AHA.112.657270.

McCall, Schell, ed. 2013. *MY Health-E-Schools,* http://crhi.org/MY-Health-e-Schools/index.html (accessed 25 March 2013).

McConnochie, Kenneth M., Conners, Gregory P., Brayer, Anne F., Goepp, Julius, Herendeen, Neil E., Wood, Nancy E., Thomas, Andrew, Ahn, Danielle S., and Roghmann, Klaus J. 2006a. "Differences in Diagnosis and Treatment Using Telemedicine Versus in-Person Evaluation of Acute Illness." *Ambulatory Pediatrics* 6, 4 (July-Aug): 187–195. doi:10.1016/j.ambp.2006.03.002.

McConnochie, Kenneth M., Conners, Gregory P., Brayer, Anne F., Goepp, Julius, Herendeen, Neil E., Wood, Nancy E., Thomas, Andrew, Ahn, Danielle S., and Roghmann, Klaus J. 2006b. "Effectiveness of Telemedicine in Replacing in-Person Evaluation for Acute Childhood Illness in Office Settings." *Telemedicine Journal and E-Health* 12, 3 (June): 308–316. doi:10.1089/tmj.2006.12.308.

McConnochie, Kenneth M., Tan, Jonathan, Wood, Nancy E., Herendeen, Neil E., Kitzman, Harriet J., Roy, Jason, and Roghmann, Klaus J. 2007. "Acute Illness Utilization Patterns Before and After Telemedicine in Childcare for Inner-City Children: A Cohort Study." *Telemedicine Journal and E-Health* 13, 4 (August): 381–390. doi:10.1089/tmj.2006.0070.

McConnochie, Kenneth M., Wood, Nancy E., Herendeen, Neil E., ten Hoopen, Cynthia B., and Roghmann, Klaus J. 2010. "Telemedicine in Urban and Suburban Childcare and Elementary Schools Lightens Family Burdens." *Telemedicine Journal and E-Health* 16, 5 (June): 533–542. doi:10.1089/tmj.2009.0138.

McGee, Meredith, and McGee, Anita. Letter. 2013. Spruce Pine, NC.

"Microwave Brings Telemedicine to Appalachia." 1976. *Emergency Medical Services* 5, 2 (March): 72–74.

Mitchell, Philip. Letter. 2013. Spruce Pine, NC.

NC Broadband. 2013. http://ncbroadband.gov/nc-recovery-projects (accessed 13 May 2013).

Pennings, Sally, and North, Steve. Letter. 2013. "Sally Pennings Telephone Interview." Saltville, VA.

Rabinowitz, Terry, Murphy, Katharine M., Amour, Judith L., Ricci, Michael A., Caputo, Michael P., and Newhouse, Paul A. 2010. "Benefits of a Telepsychiatry Consultation Service for Rural Nursing Home Residents." *Telemedicine and E-Health* 16 (1) (January): 34–40. doi:10.1089/tmj.2009.0088.

Readmissions Reduction Program. 2013. http://www.cms.gov/Medicare/Medicare-Fee-for-Service-Payment/AcuteInpatientPPS/Readmissions-Reduction-Program.html (accessed 14 May 2013).

Schweickert, Patricia A., Rutledge, Carolyn M., Cattell-Gordon, David C., Solenski, Nina J., Jensen, Mary E., Branson, Sheila, and Gaughen, John R. 2011. "Telehealth Stroke Education for Rural Elderly Virginians." *Telemedicine Journal and E-Health: The Official Journal of the American Telemedicine Association* 17, 10 (December): 784–788. doi:10.1089/tmj.2011.0080.

Silva, G.S., Farrell, S., Shandra, E., Viswanathan, A., and Schwamm, L.H. 2012. "The Status of Telestroke in the United States: a Survey of Currently Active Stroke Telemedicine Programs." *Stroke* 43 (8) (July 23): 2078–2085. doi:10.1161/STROKEAHA.111.645861.

State and County QuickFacts. 2013. United States Census Bureau, http://quickfacts.census.gov/qfd/states/37/37121.html (accessed 11 May 2013).

Telehealth Policy. 2013. National Telehealth Policy Resource Center, http://telehealth policy.us/jurisdiction/40 (accessed 23 April 2013).

Virginia's Legislative Information System. 2013. http://lis.virginia.gov/cgi-bin/legp604.exe?101+sum+SB675 (accessed 13 May 2013).

Walker, Sarah Cusworth, Kerns, Suzanne E.U., Lyon, Aaron R., Bruns, Eric J., and Cosgrove, T.J. 2010. "Impact of School-Based Health Center Use on Academic Outcomes." *Journal of Adolescent Health* 46, 3 (March): 251–257. doi:10.1016/j.jadohealth.2009.07.002.

Wampler, William. 2010. Virginia Senate Bill No. 675.

What Is Telemedicine? 2013. American Telemedicine Association, http://www.american-telemed.org/learn (accessed 7 May 2013).

Young, T.L., and Ireson, C. 2003. "Effectiveness of School-Based Telehealth Care in Urban and Rural Elementary Schools." *Pediatrics* 112, 5 (November 1): 1088–1094. doi:10.1542/peds.112.5.1088.

Mountain Empire Older Citizens, Inc., and Economic Development in Southwest Virginia: From Home-Delivered Meals to All-Inclusive Care for the Elderly

MARILYN PACE MAXWELL and TONY LAWSON

Although the economy of far southwest Virginia has been stressed for decades, the area has profited from the presence of an organization that traces its origins to the Older Americans Act and other legislation passed by Congress in 1965. The organization is Mountain Empire Older Citizens, Inc. (MEOC) and how MEOC grew over time from one person planning project into a major contributor within the local economy is the focus of this essay.

Great Society Legislation: An Introduction

American social history counts 1965 as a watershed year. It was the year that President Lyndon Baines Johnson publicized his vision of a Great Society. It was the year that America imagined a prosperous and civil nation with opportunities for all its citizens, a nation unmarred by poverty, ignorance and racial injustice. It was the year that Congress passed and President Johnson signed into law the Voting Rights Act, the Elementary and Secondary Education Act, the Older Americans Act, and the Social Security Act. These statutes came on the heels of the Civil Rights Act and the Economic Opportunity Act, both passed in 1964.

Great Society legislation authorized federal and state programs to create new economic opportunities and a social safety net for minorities; children and youth; vulnerable older citizens; and people of all ages who were struggling with poverty. Federal programs that trace their origins to 1965 include Medicare, Medicaid, Head Start, VISTA, the Job Corps, Upward Bound, the Appalachian Regional Commission and the Area Agencies on Aging. Programs authorized in 1965 have had an enormous impact on everyday life for millions of Americans — touching on education, employment, civil rights, health care and protection for ethnic minorities.

Before the expansion of the social safety net in 1965, life in America could be even more uncertain, insecure and personally frightening for millions of citizens, including many seniors. Older people had no protection against discrimination in the work place; employers could fire someone or refuse to hire someone because of age without fear of legal repercussions. Health care was not available or accessible for everyone; only those with health insurance or personal wealth enjoyed ample access to the system. Paying for medical treatment for catastrophic or chronic illness could wipe out a family's life savings and lead to bankruptcy as well as persistent poverty. With age came a whole range of new problems, including reduced income, uncertain housing, isolation and loneliness, memory loss, reduced mobility and chronic illness, all without hope of help from society at large. Individuals had to cope with age-related changes as best they could.

Life in America changed for the better with improvements contained in the Social Security Act of 1965: Medicare and Medicaid. These programs enabled older people to enjoy routine access to health care in both acute and long term settings. A third improvement came with the Older Americans Act, which enabled the creation of community-based services for older people, such as congregate and home-delivered meals, homemaker services, employment training programs and transportation.

At the signing of the Older Americans Act, President Lyndon Johnson said:

> No longer will older Americans be denied the healing miracle of modern medicine. No longer will illness crush and destroy the savings that they have so carefully put away over a lifetime so that they might enjoy dignity in their later years. No longer will young families see their own incomes, and their own hopes, eaten away simply because they are carrying out their deep moral obligations to their parents, and to their uncles, and to their aunts. And no longer will this nation refuse the hand of justice to those who have given a lifetime of service and wisdom and labor to the progress of this progressive country [http://www.presidency.ucsb.edu/ws/?pid=27079].

One of the key strategies envisioned to achieve the Great Society was the War on Poverty, the unofficial name used to describe the economic and educational reforms introduced by President Johnson in 1964. During the late 1950s and early 1960s, the American economy grew by leaps and bounds and millions of Americans prospered. Not everyone shared in the wealth though, and a portion of the population was left behind in relative poverty. By 1959, the federal government set criteria for defining poverty and started tracking the percentage of Americans deemed to be poor. That first year, the poverty rate was determined to be 22.4 percent and the nation was stunned with this news. In coming years, as news media spread the word that poverty was hidden under a prosperous veneer in America, political reformers found the widespread support they needed to reshape society.

When the federal government started tracking the poverty rate, it was clear that some sections of the country had higher rates of poverty than others. One of the regions with a disproportionately high rate of poverty was the multi-state area that stretched across the Appalachian Mountains. High unemployment and harsh living conditions during the 1950s had forced more than 2 million people in the mountains to leave their homes and seek work in other parts of the country. Of those who remained, per capita income in the region was 23 percent lower than per capita income in the United States and 33 percent of the people in Appalachia lived in poverty.

In 1960, the governors of states with territory in the eastern mountains formed a Conference of Appalachian Governors to consider ways to address economic and social problems. The governors sought help from the federal government and in 1965 Congress passed legislation that created the Appalachian Regional Commission (ARC). The purpose of the ARC was to stimulate economic development and improve the quality of life for residents of 420 counties along the spine of the Appalachian Mountains, from New York to Mississippi. The ARC has helped mountain people make better lives for themselves ever since.

The middle part of the region served by the Appalachian Regional Commission came to be called central Appalachia (for the most part Kentucky, Tennessee, West Virginia, and Virginia) and was soon famous for its coal and tobacco-producing economy — and infamous for its extraordinarily high rates of poverty. The Virginia counties of Lee, Scott and Wise and the City of Norton lie in the very heart of this central Appalachian region. These four jurisdictions create a wedge in the westernmost part of Virginia between Kentucky to the north and Tennessee to the south. They are collectively known as "far" or "extreme" southwest Virginia and they are four of the most poverty-bound communities in the state and nation.

Specific Protections for Older Appalachians

Congress passed enabling legislation for programs under the Older Americans Act in 1965, but several years went by before the programs were firmly established anywhere in the nation, including far southwest Virginia. Between 1965 and 1973, much of the work done was internal and organizational in nature, as the federal government established the Administration on Aging within the U.S. Department of Health, and then prompted the formation of State Units on Aging.

The Older Americans Act took on real significance for southwest Virginia when the Act was amended in 1973 to create local area agencies on aging. The act facilitated the establishment of area agencies on aging (AAAs) in enough local jurisdictions to serve every community in the United States.

As a result of the 1973 amendment, there are now 629 local AAAs to serve as focal points for planning, developing and rolling out services for older persons. AAAs advocate for older people in local communities by identifying needs and finding ways to address them. The agencies offer some services directly and help older people choose other home and community-based services from locally available options. AAAs help people select and preserve living arrangements that allow them to live independently as long as possible.

Over time, the national infrastructure created by the Older Americans Act came to be called the "aging network." The Older Americans Act is intentionally flexible and that flexibility permits AAAs to respond to the unique needs of older persons in their local service areas. It is often said within the aging network that if you have seen *one* area agency on aging in action, you know how *one* area agency on aging works. The Older Americans Act set the stage for Mountain Empire Older Citizens, Inc., to evolve over time, adapting services to local conditions and stimulating development in the heart of central Appalachia.

The promise of the Older Americans Act reached far southwest Virginia in late 1973 when the LENOWISCO Planning District Commission (serving Lee, Scott and Wise counties as well as the city of Norton) asked the DILENOWISCO Educational Cooperative, an agency that no longer exists, to administer a gerontology planning grant. In January 1974, DILENOWISCO hired Marilyn Pace as a regional gerontology planner and charged her with the task of developing an area plan on aging for the counties LENOWISCO served. Pace was given the task of creating an organizational structure to deliver Older Americans Act services to the people of southwest Virginia. The planning grant budget was $12,500. The project period was one year.

Community Voices:
Setting Agendas, Establishing Trust

The planner, a co-author of this essay, went to work during the first months of 1974 and convened a series of public hearings to talk about setting up a local AAA. The hearings were heavily attended and communities across the region grew hopeful and excited at the prospect of developing services for older citizens.

There were three basic ways that a local area agency on aging could be organized: as a private, nonprofit corporation; as a part of local government; or as a joint exercise of powers. Pace worked with several task forces and an advisory council to reach consensus about the best approach. The groups chose to form an independent corporation. They wanted a fresh start, an agency free from partisan politics, nepotism and other destructive forces that can plague local governments. They also wanted an agency that could act regionally and become an advocate for older persons within all levels of government. The planning groups agreed that the private, non-profit corporate structure offered the best avenue for long term success.

A few influential individuals opposed the nonprofit model, stating that the work of the new agency would duplicate efforts already underway by other organizations. The opposition soon wilted in the face of facts, though. At the time, there were no community-based long term care services for older people and their families in the targeted service area. The people who first opposed the venture quickly recanted and became strong supporters, agreeing that a new organization was exactly what the situation demanded. The independent, flexible structure of the new agency set the stage for remarkable growth in the years to come and the organization's commitment to community service turned it into an economic development engine (creating jobs, recruiting skilled workers to the region, and leveraging grants at state and federal levels) as it crafted programs and services to meet local needs and carry out its mission.

The early days of Mountain Empire Older Citizens were exciting and groundbreaking times. Public discussion of issues confronting older persons was something new, not only in rural southwest Virginia, but in most parts of the country. Older people in Appalachia who had long been silent found their voices when given an opportunity to speak. And they had plenty to say. A theme first voiced at MEOC public hearings and expressed consistently and clearly in subsequent years was the strong desire to age in place, to live at home in one's own community among family and friends while continuing to contribute to society in meaningful ways. A consistent fear expressed by older people was the dread of being placed in an institution in one's later years.

The Older Americans Act aimed to offer "a comprehensive array of community-based, long-term care services adequate to appropriately sustain older people in their communities and in their homes, including support to family members and other persons providing voluntary care to older individual needing long-term care services." The overarching goal of the Act was a good match for the needs expressed by local people during the 1974 hearings, held by the leaders who would form MEOC.

These leaders listened carefully to the voices of older persons and their families with the intention of crafting a mission to fit the local culture. In listening, they heard about a culture that values the home and family — not just a home and a nuclear family, but a network of homes for extended families and family connections situated in particular hills and hollows within the mountain landscape. Local people expressed a strong attachment to one's own place and one's own people. By "home" they meant something larger and more encompassing than casual listening might have revealed.

The leadership of the new agency decided that its mission should be to prevent the unnecessary institutionalization of older persons while helping elders remain at the heart of family life. This basic mission, consistent with the goals of the Older Americans Act has guided MEOC ever since.

Even as its leaders worked on basic organizational issues, the incipient agency started offering services to older people. The first services were home-delivered meals for homebound elders and congregate meals for more active older citizens. The first meals were delivered to frail elders in Norton by students from the Social Welfare Program at Clinch Valley College in Wise, Virginia. These early efforts were funded by the Older Americans Act.

Another valuable service was also instituted quickly in the earliest days of MEOC. During the initial public hearings about the need for an AAA, many older people spoke movingly about the fear of being unable to heat their homes in the winter. Energy prices had risen dramatically in 1973 and 1974 because of an oil embargo and subsequent energy crisis. Older people knew that they could not afford to pay their energy bills and still buy groceries, medicines, and other living expenses. Some were afraid they might not survive the winter months. Newspaper reporters wrote about the dilemma faced by older people in reams of articles and editorials and political cartoons, repeating and amplifying the theme that older people were being forced to choose between buying food or medicine and heating their homes.

Esther Congo, at that time a local businesswoman from the Town of

Wise, read the newspaper articles and was moved to action. She wanted to make sure that no older person living in the coalfields of southwest Virginia would go without food or fuel because of low income and high power bills. Congo asked other businesses for donations and appeared in the office of the gerontology planner with $900, saying, "You have got to do something. This is unacceptable. We cannot live in a place where our older friends, neighbors and relatives have to make such horrendous decisions."

In response to the fears expressed by local people and inspired by Congo's action, the agency that would become MEOC organized an Emergency Fuel Fund for the Elderly and helped people pay their fuel bills in the winter of 1974-75. The agency's quick response to the home heating needs of the local elderly population brought the new initiative widespread acceptance, approval, and support. It is not exaggerating to state that all of the work done by MEOC has been built upon the trust formed between the agency and the community through the emergency fuel campaign of 1974-75.

With the establishment of the Emergency Fuel Fund, the community realized that the new agency was truly going to respond to the expressed concerns and needs of the region's older population, rather than follow its own or a set agenda. If MEOC had not responded at this critical juncture to this critical need, the new agency may not have been so embraced by the community, but instead become just another program with high hopes and well-crafted plans that could not deliver on its promises.

Over the past 38 years, the Emergency Fuel Fund for the Elderly has evolved into a dynamic partnership of community-minded individuals, churches, health care organizations, schools, colleges, civic organizations and businesses, all committed to helping older citizens trapped in energy emergencies over the cold winter months. Led by MEOC, the community has raised more than $2.75 million and helped tens of thousands of frail, low income elders heat their homes in winter. The money is raised through local donations and fundraising events. The largest event is an annual Walkathon, held on the first Sunday in May of each year. The stated purpose of the Emergency Fuel Fund "is to help older people meet one of the most basic needs for staying healthy, safe, secure and happy — a warm home."

The Emergency Fuel Fund is raised from purely local sources and the money is returned to the economy of far southwest Virginia. All donations help older people directly; not a single penny is, or has ever been, used for salaries, office supplies, or anything other than paying the fuel bills of older people in need. Everyone who contributes to the Emergency Fuel Fund relies on this knowledge and trusts the proven stewardship of MEOC.

Recognizing early that trust is difficult to gain, easy to lose, and hard to repair if broken, MEOC learned early to value this intangible asset; thus subsequent planning and programming has followed this listening pattern.

MEOC relies on local funding to support its programs. In 2011, local contributors gave $530,000 to MEOC, while local governments added another $179,800. Of the $530,000 sub-total, $222,000 was designated for the Emergency Fuel Fund. In the winter of 2011-12, the Emergency Fuel Fund helped 1,118 frail and needy older citizens stay warm. Echoes of the voices of the frightened elders who first spoke about their fears in 1974 can still be heard every winter in far southwest Virginia.

Far southwest Virginia's gerontology planning initiative was at first part of the DILENOWISCO Educational Cooperative. The initiative re-invented itself, after a time of careful planning, into a non-profit organization and submitted its articles of incorporation to the Commonwealth of Virginia on August 31, 1976. With an eight-member Board of Directors and a fifty-member Advisory Council, Mountain Empire Older Citizens, Inc., set out in the fall of 1976 to fulfill the promises and dreams of the Older Americans Act in rural southwest Virginia. Thirty-six years later, MEOC remains faithful to its core mission, shaped in response to local voices heard in 1974: to help older people live in their own homes and communities and avoid being placed in institutions unless absolutely necessary. MEOC has crafted many programs around this core mission and has extended the age range of clients served in order because older people do not live in a vacuum; services that benefit other age groups also benefit them. MEOC has devoted almost four decades to providing community based services that support older people living at home, as well as the extended families that take care of them.

Here is the current MEOC mission statement:

Mountain Empire Older Citizens, Inc. is committed to the prevention of unnecessary and/or inappropriate institutionalization of older persons by: the development and maintenance of comprehensive user-friendly community based long term care services in Lee, Wise, Scott Counties, and the City of Norton; recognizing that families provide the bulk of care for older people and then developing a user-friendly comprehensive infrastructure to support family caregivers; and by serving as an active and responsible advocate on issues effecting older persons; and

Mountain Empire Older Citizens, Inc. is further committed to the concept of intergenerational programming and is devoted to developing programs utilizing the talents and skills of both the young and the old in service to each other and by supporting relatives caring for children other than their own; and

Mountain Empire Older Citizens, Inc. strongly believes that healthy people and healthy families result in healthy communities and works to achieve this. Thus, MEOC emphasizes wellness and health promotion as part of its mission to promote a quality life for all. Physical health, mental health, economic security, spirituality, and emotional health are all important, interrelated aspects of true wellness; and

Mountain Empire Older Citizens, Inc. is committed to developing and maintaining a specialized and public transportation system that is for all ages, all clients and patients of area health and human services organizations and which is seamless and coordinated; and

Mountain Empire Older Citizens, Inc. is committed to the prevention of abuse of both the young and the old, to protecting the rights of all ages in harmful and potentially harmful situations, and to supporting families in ways to promote safe and healthy homes; and

Mountain Empire Older Citizens, Inc. is committed to carrying out its mission in partnership with our local community and those individuals, organizations, and agencies sharing similar goals and values who demonstrate the ability to work together in a truly collaborative manner. This partnership of families and communities is central to all of the efforts of Mountain Empire Older Citizens, Inc. [www.meoc.org].

In 1999, MEOC was prompted to re-examine and expand its mission when a community coalition concerned with child abuse prevention, intervention and treatment asked MEOC to administer a Healthy Families Program. In 2000 MEOC set up a regional Children's Advocacy Center to serve and treat victims of child abuse. At about the same time, MEOC care coordinators noticed that more and more grandparents were raising their grandchildren because the parents were absent or incapacitated. In response, MEOC developed a KinCare program to support grandparents and other caregivers who serve as surrogate parents for related children.

To administer these new initiatives, MEOC created a Department of Children's Services, a unique move among area agencies on aging. The new division included KinCare, the southwest Virginia Children's Advocacy Center, and Healthy Families of southwest Virginia. By expanding its vision to help the children of families in dire straits, MEOC brought to the region unique financial resources to address problems that beset extended families in this corner of Virginia.

In 2002, MEOC began providing management services to the Junction Center for Independent Living (JCIL). JCIL is a non-profit organization that helps people with significant disabilities to live in the least restrictive, most integrated setting possible. The JCIL mission for people with disabilities mirrors the MEOC mission for older persons. Both agencies preserve the independence of people at risk of institutional placement. MEOC and JCIL share a staff person and are partners in the Aging and Disabilities Resource Center and Pharmacy Connect of southwest Virginia.

The MEOC-JCIL decision to collaborate proved to be prophetic, anticipating state and federal moves to consolidate the aging network with the disabilities network. In 2012, Virginia combined the Department for the Aging and the Department of Rehabilitative Services to create a new Department of Aging and Rehabilitative Services. Also in 2012, the federal government created a new administration to fund and oversee programs for older persons and those with significant disabilities.

While announcing the new federal division on April 6, 2012, United States Secretary of Health and Human Services Kathleen Sebelius said that the Administration for Community Living combines "the Administration on Aging, the Office on Disability and the Administration on Developmental Disabilities into a single agency that supports both cross-cutting initiatives and efforts focused on the unique needs of individual groups such as children with developmental disabilities or seniors with dementia. This new agency will work on increasing access to community supports and achieving full community participation for people" (leadingage.org).

As suggested by the MEOC-JCIL alliance, MEOC is guided by a philosophy of asset-based community development. The organization does not focus on the scarcity of resources in central Appalachia or bewail the region's poverty, lack of infrastructure, high unemployment and low educational attainment. Rather, MEOC identifies existing resources and assets within the region and builds on them through collaboration with state and federal sources, the private sector and the religious community to create new opportunities for growth and development. MEOC is a mission-driven organization that identifies local needs and then responds to them with fitting strategies, using local assets and partnerships as well as resources available through larger state and national communities.

Since volunteers first delivered meals to older individuals in Norton in 1974, MEOC has refined and expanded its services many times to include new programs and serve additional clients. The agency's strategy has been to build an infrastructure of community-based services that enables older persons and their families to live at home in health, honor and dignity. Today, there is increased emphasis within the aging network on the idea of "aging in place," a concept articulated by hundreds of older southwest Virginians way back in 1974. The desire to age in place has grown stronger and deeper each year since and still guides MEOC in its decisions, actions and service offerings.

As examples of listening-to-the-community-responsiveness, two of the largest departments within MEOC — Mountain Empire Transit and the Mountain Empire Program of All-Inclusive Care for the Elderly (PACE) are covered below in some detail. Along with the MEOC Department of Family Support Services, these departments employ a large percentage of MEOC's 300 plus employees. It is through the operation of these three departments that MEOC exerts its greatest influence on the local economy.

MEOC anticipated the centrifugal forces that can separate departments and create silos within large agencies, and avoided such pitfalls by assigning to staff tasks that cross department boundaries. MEOC's management team is also composed of all the department heads, and the team meets and communicates regularly. The overarching message and core strength of this approach is that the whole is greater than the sum of its parts.

The following list of service offered at MEOC hints at the variety of ways the agency supports older persons and their families. (The list does not include children's services.) For more information and an explanation of each of service, visit the agency web site at www.meoc.org.

- Adult Day Health Care — Two centers
- Care Coordination and Transitions
- Congregate Nutrition Program — Nine centers
- Emergency Services
- The Senior Community Service Employment Program (often referred to as Title V Older Workers' Program)
- Home Delivered Meals (often referred to as Meals on Wheels)
- Homemaker Services
- In-home Respite Services
- Information and Assessment
- Mountain Laurel Cancer Resource and Support Center
- Legal Services
- Aging and Disabilities Resource Center
- Personal Care Services
- Pharmacy Connect of Southwest Virginia
- Volunteer Insurance Counseling and Assistance Program
- Personal Emergency Response Services
- Senior Farmers' Market Nutrition Program
- Alzheimer's Family Support Services
- "Cancer: Surviving and Thriving" Workshops
- Chronic Disease Self-Management Program Workshops
- Elder Abuse Prevention Services
- Faith Works Partnership
- Public Guardianship Program
- Long Term Care Ombudsman
- Foster Grandparents Program
- Public Information and Education

- Kinship Care Services for older relatives raising children of family members
- Public and Specialized Transportation Services
- Volunteer Driver Program
- Transit Mobility Management Services
- Program of All-Inclusive Care for the Elderly

Evolution of Mountain Empire Transit

One of the fundamental ways that MEOC supports the local economy is through the provision of coordinated transportation services. From its earliest days, MEOC recognized the importance of reliable transportation. The public hearings held in 1974 revealed that a lack of transportation was a major barrier to social services for older people and in rural southwest Virginia. More formal needs assessments and conversations with elected officials and providers of health and human services underscored the problem. MEOC realized that the agency had to create access to affordable transportation in order to run programs in a distressed rural area.

With its first congregate meals program in 1974, MEOC began providing transportation for its clientele, driving older people between their homes and the nutrition sites, with occasional trips for shopping. It was a limited service, but an important first step in gaining experience in the field of transportation. MEOC received funding from the Tennessee Valley Authority to buy its first van and the agency bought more vehicles as new funding opportunities came available.

One of the objectives of the Older Americans Act was to promote readily available, low cost transportation so that older people could choose living arrangements and get whatever services they needed across a broad continuum of care. MEOC committed itself to the development of a coordinated transportation system for far southwest Virginia, one that would facilitate access to health care as well as social and consumer services.

While the Older Americans Act promoted transportation, it did not fully finance the service. As MEOC grew, the need for reliable transportation outpaced dollars available from the Older Americans Act, so the organization started looking for ways to finance and develop a new, larger system. As a first step, MEOC canvassed health and human services organizations in the region to discuss transportation issues, and quickly learned that almost every organization was struggling to deliver its own services to people who lived outside the boundaries of the small towns and coal camps in the area.

Each agency was trying to address the transportation problem and each agency was failing. It was a sincere but fragmented approach.

MEOC convened a series of planning meetings with these other agencies to explore the issues further. MEOC had created flexible routes to transport clients to/from its congregate meal sites and other programs. Similarly, other agencies had worked out transportation routes to make sure their clients could access services. Several agencies decided to join with MEOC and coordinate transportation routes to more efficiently pick up and deliver clients for services. MEOC assumed a leadership role and began working on a plan to meet the combined transportation needs of all the participating organizations. By 1985, MEOC had created a coordinated transportation system that served clients of several human services agencies and had the capacity to bring other agencies into the system, so the organization approached the Virginia Department of Rail and Public Transportation with a plan to open agency transport services to all citizens, thereby creating a badly-needed regional public transportation system for the region. The Department of Rail and Public Transportation supported the plan and contracted with MEOC to provide transportation for the general public.

Re-developing its transportation system to accommodate the public was a pivotal step in the evolution of MEOC. The agency christened the new service "Mountain Empire Transit." In 1988 MEOC obtained funding to hire a full-time Transit Director and purchase additional buses. Since 1988, the Transit system has grown with the times. Today, Mountain Empire Transit has a budget of $2.1 million. MEOC employs 61 drivers, dispatchers and administrative staff and uses 72 vehicles to provide about 115,000 trips a year. In fiscal year 2011, Mountain Empire Transit served 2,722 unduplicated people.

The transit system is housed in a separate building on the MEOC campus. Completed in 2005, the building covers 9,900 square feet and includes offices, meeting space, a dispatch center and several maintenance bays. Building and furnishing the building cost $1.45 million. Grant funds for the project came from the Federal Transit Administration.

Thus Mountain Empire Transit has grown into a model transit system for rural communities. In 2008 MEOC received the United We Ride Leadership Award presented by the United States Secretary of Transportation Ray LaHood. The award recognized Mountain Empire Transit for effective public transit and human services transportation coordination, planning and implementation. The award affirmed the success of MEOC's commitment to bring a unified health and human services transportation system to the mountains of central Appalachia. This national recognition was preceded in 2004 by the Federal Transit Administration Administrator's Award for Outstanding Public Service. MEOC received that award for "success in enhancing the mobility of rural residents through the coordination of services and multiple funding sources."

Mountain Empire Transit continues to seek better and more creative ways to serve the citizens of far southwest Virginia. Ready access to an integrated and coordinated public and health and human services transportation system makes it feasible for MEOC to serve eligible people with a broad array of services. The organization could never have developed congregate nutrition sites, adult day health care centers, community group respite centers or the PACE program without having Mountain Empire Transit already in place.

Development of Mountain Empire PACE

In 1996, MEOC started to explore the idea of launching a Program of All Inclusive Care for the Elderly (PACE). PACEs are managed care organizations that contract with Medicare and Medicaid to provide services for older adults with chronic illnesses. PACE provides services to those who need long term help with the activities of daily living, such as dressing, bathing, walking and toileting. PACE organizations provide care in a community setting and offer an alternative to the placement of frail elders in nursing facilities.

PACE is a specific model of healthcare whose origin can be traced to an innovative adult day health center in a multicultural community in San Francisco in 1973. The adult day health center was called On Lok, which means "peaceful, happy abode" in Cantonese. Starting as a simple senior center, On Lok added services in piecemeal fashion over a five year period in order to meet needs expressed by older residents in the community, including medical services, home health, personal care, transportation, and rehabilitation.

In 1979, On Lok received a four year grant from the Department of Health and Human Services (DHHS) to create a consolidated model for delivering acute and long term care to older people in a community setting. In 1983, DHHS authorized On Lok to test prospective payment for integrated acute and long term care, a system called "capitation." In this system, On Lok received a set monthly payment from Medicare and Medicaid for each person enrolled in the program. In return, On Lok provided a broad array of health and social services.

In 1986, federal law extended On Lok's capitation system to other agencies and allowed 10 organizations in cities across the country to replicate On Lok's service delivery and funding model. In 1990, DHHS awarded Medicare and Medicaid waivers to all 11 programs and gave them the name "Program of All Inclusive Care for the Elderly."

A Program of All Inclusive Care for the Elderly (PACE) is a managed care plan that enrolls frail seniors and provides them with health and social services designed to keep them living safely at home as long as possible. Seniors enroll in the PACE plan and receive care under the guidance of an interdisciplinary team of healthcare professionals. Participants receive medical, nursing, pharmacy, nutrition, recreation, personal care, social services, rehabilitation and transportation in an adult day care setting that is enhanced with primary care and restorative clinics. Core services — adult day care, primary medical care and rehabilitation — are provided at a central location called the PACE Center. Other services are provided in the homes of program participants or in hospitals, nursing facilities or doctors' offices.

PACE plans offer insurance coverage for every service covered under Medicare and Medicaid, including specialty medical care, hospitalization, prescription drugs, lab, x-ray and diagnostic services, skilled nursing and long-term custodial care. PACE plans may choose to cover additional items as well, such as dental care, vision and hearing services or home modifications.

The PACE model was established as a permanent type of healthcare provider in the Balanced Budget Act of 1997. Although it was possible to set up a PACE organization anywhere in the nation after 1997, PACE remained an urban model of care for the next decade. New programs were opened almost exclusively by large health systems in major cities.

Since the object of PACE is consistent with the original mission of MEOC and the Older Americans Act, MEOC turned its attention to creating one. Originally, the board was inclined to create a Program of All-Inclusive Care for the Elderly in partnership with a local hospital. MEOC staff and board members visited PACE organizations in Baltimore, Maryland and Columbia, South Carolina and witnessed firsthand the capacity of PACE to provide everything frail older people need to live well in their own homes and communities.

However, the hospital in mind dropped out of the partnership plan and MEOC decided to await future opportunities for developing the project. That opportunity appeared in 2006 when Congress appropriated $7.5 million for the Centers for Medicare and Medicaid Services (CMS) to make grants to rural organizations that wanted to set up the PACE model. MEOC applied for a federal grant and received $500,000 in start-up funds, the maximum available. That same year, Virginia decided to support PACE and awarded grants of $250,000 to five nonprofit organizations across the state. MEOC received both state and federal grants and accrued enough capital to pursue the project.

Becoming a PACE organization is an expensive, time-consuming proposition. Preparing an application and securing approval from Medicaid and Medicare requires the oversight of a determined planner and usually takes more than a year to complete. Applicant agencies must describe in detail how every single service covered by Medicare and Medicare can be supplied to local program participants in every part of its targeted service area. The detailed plans must be presented first to the state Medicaid agency for criticism and approval and then to Medicare for further refinement. Medicaid and Medicare take six to nine months to review and approve applications.

Meanwhile, the potential PACE organization must prepare a separate proposal to become a Medicare Part D sponsor and prepare a detailed bid to offer prescription medications to program clientele. Medicare Part D is a complex program and preparing a bid requires the services of an actuarial accountant to assess financial risks, predict utilization rates and forecast a reliable profit/loss scenario. While the application process is underway, the organization must build and equip a PACE Center and obtain approval from local and state authorities to use the space as an adult day care center, medical clinic and rehabilitation treatment facility. The facility must be turn-key ready to operate before Medicare and Medicaid will finally approve the application. Because a PACE organization must prepare a facility to meet exacting standards well in advance of providing reimbursable services, the organization needs access to considerable capital.

Moreover, before Medicare and Medicaid will approve a PACE start-up, the applicant agency must hire and train a full complement of professionals and be ready to provide services to the first cadre of participants enrolled in the health plan. This means that months before the agency is paid to provide care, it must have professional staff, including a program director, physician, registered nurse and clinical team, adult day care center manager, masters level social worker, registered dietitian, physical therapist, recreation therapist, home care coordinator, occupational therapist, transportation coordinator, van drivers and personal care aides.

These professionals must be trained to function as an interdisciplinary team, a panel at the heart of the PACE model of care. Many health professionals are trained to work within a rigid hierarchy, with physicians at the top and every other discipline in a supporting role. In contrast, the PACE model contends that every member of the interdisciplinary team holds valuable information about participants, information to which no other team member has access, so each team member must be respected and empowered to share information in a supportive setting.

The interdisciplinary team serves multiple roles in the PACE model. Individuals on the team provide many health and social services directly to participants. The team also plans, arranges and facilitates the provision of services purchased from external contractors on behalf of participants. The team is the authorizer of services, deciding what is medically necessary for the continued wellbeing of each participant.

PACE organizations are not just service providers; they are also insurance plans. Each PACE must either manage a claims adjudication system or contract with a third party administrator to adjudicate and pay claims from hospitals, doctors and other health care providers. Likewise, each PACE must either manage its own Part D insurance plan or contract with a pharmacy benefits manager to facilitate this branch of Medicare, which pays for prescription drugs. Finally, each PACE must contract with a network of health care providers to assure access to every covered service on behalf of patients who enroll in the program.

MEOC contracted with an experienced PACE executive from Columbia, South Carolina to write its original grant application to CMS for Rural PACE start-up funds in 2005/2006. MEOC then contracted with Palmetto Senior Care, a technical assistance agency in Columbia to obtain some templates for a provider package and develop a five year financial pro forma. MEOC employed a PACE Director in February 2007 and the agency submitted its provider application to Virginia Medicaid between April and June of that year. Medicaid approved the application in July 2007 and forwarded it to Medicare for review.

Medicare considered the proposal for 90 days and requested additional information in October 2007. MEOC adjusted the plans to meet Medicare requirements and re-submitted in November 2007. Virginia Medicaid completed a readiness review of the space renovated for PACE within the MEOC headquarters in October 2007 and pronounced the facility ready to operate. Medicare reviewed the program application for an additional 90 days and then issued a letter approving MEOC as a permanent PACE provider on February 6, 2008. By February 15, 2008, MEOC, Medicaid and Medicare had signed a three way agreement that created Mountain Empire PACE and permitted the program to start recruiting participants.

MEOC had employed a center manager in October 2007 and a medical director in January 2008. The rest of the professional team came aboard on Valentine's Day, February 14, 2008, and the new program enrolled its first set of participants on April 1, 2008.

Two people enrolled on that date. It was an inauspicious beginning, but PACE grew quickly, with eleven more participants enrolled in May, seven in June. The program census reached 40 by December 2008.

When Mountain Empire PACE opened, the program was housed in about 3,500 square feet of space within the MEOC headquarters building. The space had been renovated and furnished while the application process was still underway. The initial PACE Center was licensed to have a maximum of 38 participants on the premises at any given time. Not every participant attends the PACE Center every day, so the limit of 38 individuals per day meant that Mountain Empire PACE could enroll a total of 70–75 participants before needing more space.

MEOC planned for PACE to outgrow its initial quarters. The agency described its long term plans for PACE to the Wise County Industrial Development Authority and in 2006, the Wise County IDA donated a piece of real estate to MEOC for construction of the PACE Center. The land was valued at $75,000 and located on a mountainside across the street from MEOC headquarters.

With a building site in place, MEOC applied to the Virginia Tobacco Indemnification and Community Revitalization Commission (Tobacco Commission) for a grant to use in hiring an architect to construct a new PACE Center. The Tobacco Commission recognized the economic development potential for Mountain Empire PACE and in 2006 awarded a grant of $162,500 to MEOC for the project. MEOC hired an architect who presented the agency with a set of drawings and specifications in April 2007. The plans called for construction of a single story structure covering 17,023 square feet.

With a building site and construction plans now in place, MEOC applied to the Department of Agriculture Office of Rural Development (USDA) for a low interest loan to build a new PACE Center. USDA issued a long list of terms and conditions that MEOC had to meet before soliciting construction bids and breaking ground. MEOC completed the last of the loan terms and conditions in November 2007 and authorized the architect to advertise in local papers for construction bids in January 2008. A bid conference was held in February 2008 and the contract was awarded to a local company, Quesenberry's, Inc. MEOC held a ground-breaking ceremony for the new building on May 20, 2008 and was honored by the presence of then–Virginia Governor Timothy Kaine and a number of elected officials and administrators from state and local agencies. Construction started in May 2008 and ended in December 2009, when Mountain Empire PACE occupied the new building. By that time, the program's census had grown to 61.

A key component of PACE is the development of a contracted network of healthcare providers to meet the needs of participants in the program. As a provider of long term care services intended to help older citizens preserve their independence, MEOC already had in place several key components of a provider network. MEOC offered social service referrals, case management, transportation, congregate and home delivered meals, home-based personal care, homemaker services, companion care, group and emergency respite care, caregiver support programs, adult protective services, a personal alarm service and a guardianship program. MEOC also had years of experience in operating adult day healthcare centers. But between March 2007 and April 2008, Mountain Empire PACE created a healthcare provider network to complement the MEOC system of community-based social services. Key components of the network fell into place when two major hospital systems in the region agreed to work with the new program. With the support of these hospitals, MEOC recruited a broad array of medical specialists and other healthcare providers to participate in the network. After a surge of contractual activity between January and March 2008, the Mountain Empire PACE network included 200 health service providers in southwest Virginia and northeast Tennessee. Within a few years, the number of contracted partners in the system exceeded 250.

The MEOC fiscal year runs from October 1st through September 30th. In the six months between the PACE start date on April 1 (PACE has always been one to attract good dates; after all we hired our care team on Valentine's Day) and the end of its first fiscal year on September 30, MEOC employed a total of 24 people in full-time or part-time positions for PACE. The PACE portion of the payroll was $0.47 million for this period and the program spent $0.23 million on the purchase of health and social services from other providers. Total expenses for the program amounted to $0.85 million in its first six months of operation.

Mountain Empire PACE grew substantially the next year. By September 2009, enrollment had climbed to 58 participants and there were 44 employees on the payroll. For the fiscal year that ended on September 30, 2009, the PACE portion of the MEOC payroll was $1.20 million and the amount spent by Mountain Empire PACE on the purchase of other health and social services for participants was $2.03 million. Total expenses came to $3.51 million for the year.

In September 2010, PACE enrollment stood at 71 and the program employed 55 full-time or part-time staff. Expenses for the year totaled $5.04 million, with a payroll of $1.51 million and purchased health and social services valued at $3.23 million. During this critical year, MEOC had to flex its financial muscle to cover expenses for the PACE operation. Expenses for Mountain Empire PACE exceeded revenue by almost half a million dollars that year.

Effective management, increased enrollment, and staff changes improved the situation for the year that ended in September 2011. By that time, enrollment had increased to 92 and the program employed 51 fulltime or part-time staff. The payroll was $1.64 million and the cost of purchasing other health and social services for participants amounted to $3.65 million. Expenses for the year amounted to $5.73 million and program revenue exceeded expenses by more $0.8 million.

Mountain Empire PACE enrollment climbed to 100 in December 2011 and then fluctuated between 96 and 100 for the first six months of 2012 before reaching 105 in August. Expenses for the first nine months of the fiscal year that began October 1, 2011, were $4.68 million, with $1.42 million in payroll and $2.83 million in network payments. MEOC employs 56 fulltime or part-time workers to staff the program.

In other words, PACE became not just a needed service for the elderly in our community, but an economic development powerhouse, not only creating jobs for skilled health care workers, but enabling those with no one to look after elderly loved ones by day to go out and work with the assurance that their family members were being looked after in a state-of-the-art facility. All of this was done by, for, and within the three far southwestern counties of Virginia.

MEOC's Growth and Economic Impact in the Community

MEOC started with one gerontology planner in 1974. The MEOC staff in 2013 includes 345 salaried and hourly employees. Included in this total are 15 enrollees in the Senior Community Services Employment Program and 30 in the Foster Grandparents Program. MEOC ranks among the larger employers in the area. Payroll for the 2011/2012 fiscal year was $6,758,984, a 12 percent increase over the previous year.

The MEOC operating budget for the 2011/2012 fiscal year was $12.6 million, a far cry from the 1974 budget of $12,500. The size of its budget and staff makes MEOC a positive influence on the region's economy. With the development of MEOC's Mountain Empire Program of All-Inclusive Care for the Elderly (PACE Program) in 2008, MEOC's economic impact increased substantially, not only in the employment arena, but in the amount of new money it circulates among MEOC's many contractors in the region. As the PACE Program continues to grow, MEOC's impact on the local economy will continue to increase.

MEOC has grown from an organization completely funded by the Older Americans Act to an organization whose appropriations from the Older Americans Act now total only 9 percent of MEOC's operating budget and that percentage decreases yearly. The following analysis of the agency's 2011 budget indicates the sources of revenue for MEOC programs.

Revenue Source	Amount	Percent of Budget
Virginia Department of Medical Assistance Services	$ 3,513,974	28%
Center for Medicare and Medicaid Services	$ 3,312,274	28%
Virginia Department for the Aging State and Federal	$ 2,150,982	17%
Department of Rail and Public Transportation	$ 1,316,876	10%
Virginia Department of Social Services	$ 243,231	2%
Federal "Stimulus" ARRA	$ 286,909	4%
Fees for Services	$ 510,701	4%
Transportation Contract Services Revenues	$ 345,533	3%
Corporation for National Service	$ 148,091	1%
Local Governments and Local Contracts	$ 277,947	2%
Local Fundraising	$ 529,470	4%

MEOC has benefited several times from the unwavering support of the Wise County Industrial Development Authority (Wise County IDA). The Wise County IDA has consistently appreciated the value of MEOC as an economic engine for the region; donated land to MEOC; and issued bonds to raise money to construct MEOC facilities and to expand the agency's campus.

MEOC first approached the Wise County IDA in 1989 to ask for assistance in constructing an office complex. The Wise County IDA donated land to MEOC in the Big Stone Gap Industrial Park and underwrote an Industrial Revenue Bond to construct the agency's first office building. The building covered 7,065 square feet and cost $350,000. MEOC moved to its new facility in late 1990. With the new office space, MEOC services grew dramatically and the agency employed many more people. By 1999, the growing agency needed additional space, so the Wise County IDA issued a second Industrial Revenue Bond to expand the size of the 1990 office building. The expansion covered 11,000 square feet and cost $1.1 million.

This is significant in light of the fact that action taken by the Wise County Industrial Development Authority brought some criticism. Some residents of the Big Stone Gap area questioned the wisdom of assisting a private, nonprofit human services agency. The critics thought that the property used for MEOC should have been preserved in the hope of recruiting a "real" business to provide "real" jobs. The Wise County IDA showed great foresight in supporting MEOC, as the figures above show, and its support has enabled MEOC to be a consistent creator of jobs in the community for decades. Just 38 years after the $12,500 gerontology planning grant that created it, local economic development leaders estimate that the economic value of MEOC doing business in far southwest Virginia in Fiscal year 2011 was $17.6 million. The support of the Wise County Industrial Development Authority continues to be essential to the continued development of MEOC. On several occasions when MEOC has needed capital in order to develop new programs and employ more workers, the Wise County IDA has helped the agency obtain the necessary funding.

Thirty-eight years following the delivery of its first service in 1974, MEOC ranks among the largest employers in far southwest Virginia. The Virginia Employment Commission's Quarterly Census of Employment and Wages for the last quarter of 2011 lists Mountain Empire Older Citizens as 17th on the list of the region's 50 Largest Employers. Given MEOC's projected continued growth, the organization anticipates moving upward on that list each year.

The story of MEOC's birth and development holds many smaller stories, but the baseline is that everything MEOC did was based on first listening to the community and responding to its need; all the economic benefits that came later stemmed from sincere efforts to improve the quality of life in southwest Virginia for a substantial number of its residents. MEOC has given many older persons the opportunity to age in place at home among family and friends. In Fiscal Year 2011, MEOC's services directly assisted 12,600 persons. That number increases yearly. Mountain Empire Older Citizens, Inc. intends to continue meeting the needs of southwest Virginia's growing population of older adults, all the while being one of the region's best employers and greatest success stories.

References

Johnson, Lyndon B. 1965. "Remarks at the Signing of the Older Americans Act." http://www.presidency.ucsb.edu/ws/?pid=27079.

Mountain Empire Older Citizens website. http://www.meoc.org/.

Sebelius, Kathleen. 2012. Announcement on Administration for Community Living. April 6, http://www.leadingage.org/HHS_Launches_Administration_for_Community_Living.aspx.

PART THREE: CULTURAL THEORY AND CLINICAL POLICY

The Elephant on the Examining Table: "Patient Responsibility" Examined as a Construct of Public Health and Clinical Health Care

WENDY WELCH and ESTHER THATCHER, RN

The concepts of responsibility and cultural competency have major impacts on how we provide care to individuals, families, and communities. This essay describes personal and corporate responsibility, and how it interacts with culture in providing health services in Appalachia.

Personal Responsibility

The Oxford English Dictionary defines responsibility as "the capability of fulfilling an obligation or duty; the state or fact of being accountable; liability, accountability *for* something." Personal and patient are terms with commonly accepted definitions; thus we can take "personal/patient responsibility" to literally mean that a person who is undergoing some form of care accepts a duty and accountability toward his or her conduct.

Personal responsibility is a concept that often enters the patient-provider relationship when providers judge the cause of a health problem to be rooted in the patient's own behavior or choices. For example, obesity is often viewed as a result of an individual's sloth and gluttony: too little exercise and too much food. Likewise, Type II diabetes, heart disease, hypertension, osteoarthritis, and other diseases linked to obesity are seen as preventable if the patient had taken better care of themselves. Thus, when health care providers judge a health problem to be the result of patients abdicating responsibility for their own well-being, a sense of justice may ask why scarce health care resources should be used to compensate for this personal irresponsibility.

Many of the reasons for these judgments are linked to deeply embedded traits of Western and Christian cultures. Since the time of Plato and Aristotle, the virtues of *prudence, justice, fortitude,* and *temperance* have remained key elements of moral excellence (Hughes 1998). Early Christians solidified the list of "seven deadly sins": *pride, envy, wrath, greed, lust, sloth* and *gluttony* (Dietz 2008). The phrase "God helps those who help themselves" is representative of the pervasive idea that individuals who show the initiative to take care of themselves deserve more mercy than those who do not.

Patient responsibility (used interchangeably with the term "personal responsibility" in this essay) is often employed when discussing health concerns perceived to have some element of personal behavior involved in their onset. These include Type II diabetes, heart disease, hypertension and other conditions associated with obesity; substance abuse, including prescription drug misuse, street drugs, alcohol and the related health issues of injuries and mental health disorders; sexually transmitted infections; and tobacco use, including lung cancer, respiratory infections, cardiovascular disease, and related issues.

Health problems believed to be caused by individual behavior carry a stigma that reflects the societal value of taking personal responsibility for one's health (DeJong 1993; Puhl & Heuer 2010). As an interesting side note, several research approaches show that stigmatization tends to have multiple negative effects on individual and public health, particularly in cases of obesity, but also in diseases such as HIV/AIDS and tuberculosis (Puhl & Heuer 2010). Put simply, stigmas actually worsen the health problems that they condemn.

The tendency to place blame on the patient for certain diseases is complicated by several factors. First is the cases of these diseases in patients who do not match the stereotypical profile. For example, between 10 and 15 percent of lung cancers occur in people who do not smoke (Brody 2010), and Type II diabetes can affect people who are underweight. But the concept of personal responsibility associated with behavior causing illness, particularly chronic illness, is still applied in implicit and overt ways.

The center of the argument for individuals to take personal responsibility for their health is that a behavior the individual is engaged in must have a causal role in some undesirable outcome, and this causal role must be known. There must be agreed-upon standards to judge the outcome, as well as a method for judging it. Finally, the individual must have a choice of alternate behaviors. For example, there is considerable scientific evidence that smoking can cause lung cancer. If an individual chooses to smoke, or to be around second-hand smoke, then he or she is seen as having at least a partial causal role in the undesirable outcome of lung cancer. Despite the science of causation, these criteria of responsibility are open to individual judgment; what looks impossible to one person may look like the road not taken, perhaps out of apathy or laziness, to another (Frolich et al., 2001).

Personal responsibility may be emerging as central to twenty-first century health policy, but its roots go back to Nixon's presidency, and the formation and current shape of today's insurance industry. As early as 1974, insurance companies used personal responsibility when outlining their policies, not only for pricing coverage but also denying claims (Bickelhaupt 1974). Insurance and other healthcare financing programs have since that time increasingly used the patient responsibility when determining eligibility and benefits (Blacksher 2008; Hermer 2008) and particularly in policies pertaining to chronic health issues associated with obesity (Kersh 2009; Brownell et al., 2010).

Patient responsibility can be divided into a forward-looking and retrospective approach within the insurance milieu. Forward-looking responsibility seeks to prevent health problems by encouraging individual behavior and choices that are good for the self, others, and the healthcare system (Schmidt 2009). In this definition, Schmidt does not discuss that what is "good" for the individual, others, and the healthcare system may not be synonymous, or even have significant overlap, but he does point out that the person receiving care must have enough understanding (health literacy) to make an informed decision. In other words, accountability can only be applied if the person is free to make a good choice in the first place. This becomes a critical point when discussing patient responsibility's interaction with cultural competency, as will be discussed shortly.

By contrast, retrospective responsibility holds an individual accountable for a negative outcome that has built over time through the patient's actions, perhaps despite warnings from health professionals. Obesity, tobacco-related illnesses, and substance abuse issues are the most obvious, but bear in mind that this concept depends on results over time. A person abusing a substance may make a mistake in dosage and have a heart attack the first time she takes medications not prescribed to her; this is an immediate consequence, and while it is the result of a personal choice, it is not retrospective responsibility because of its immediacy. Taken one step further, a person may eat one serving of ice cream without necessarily sliding into a pattern, but when the behavior of the individual repeats and over the course of months and years contributes to a slow slide into ill health due to a high body mass index, this is considered by health care professionals and insurers alike as retrospective. It is also almost uniformly considered personal responsibility denied.

In insurance venues, punishments for denied retrospective responsibility are finding an increasing foothold in a U.S. population concerned about escalating care costs, not least because fully one-third of Americans are now obese (National Institute of Diabetes and Digestive and Kidney Diseases, or NIDDK 2010). It is interesting to note that personal responsibility tends to outweigh corporate responsibility in such matters. As an example, in 2003, the House of Representatives considered the "Personal Responsibility in Food Consumption Act." This act limited class action lawsuits against fast food companies and other "unhealthy" food providers by individuals suffering ill health as a result of consuming them (H.R. Rep. No. 108-432, 2003). Perhaps this echoes late twentieth-century legal wrangles regarding tobacco use, when class action suits were diverted into the creation of the Tobacco Indemnification Commission (TIC). The TIC funds significant health initiatives throughout areas where tobacco is popular as both a crop and a product. A trade has been effected; these regions benefit from what one health organization availing itself of TIC funds called "blood money," but citizens who have been harmed by smoking cannot bring class action suits against tobacco companies for ill health effects.

In short, personal responsibility has been used to set policies regarding healthcare financing, to frame health intervention models, and to create (intentionally or perhaps by unexamined assumption) the value structures of healthcare providers and patients. It has also been used specifically to limit concepts of corporate responsibility.

Corporate Responsibility

The first problem concepts of patient responsibility raise is this limitation of corporate or "source" responsibility in favor of a mentality that some claim blames the victim. In the smoking lawsuits, citizens basically claimed they were not fully informed of the hazards of smoking. Secondhand smoke victims claimed they were subjected to harm which they did not choose. Tobacco companies claimed that individuals had made their own choices. Such issues remain unresolved; for all legal challenges continue to the "no more class actions" ban, questions of personal, corporate and in some cases societal responsibility also continue in legislation requesting "sin tax" and in the refusal of health insurance by private companies to individuals who smoke.

Consider another issue of personal versus corporate responsibility: eating fast food. In 2003, New Yorkers Ashley Pelman (14) and Jazlyn Bradley (19), brought suit against McDonald's, blaming the fast-food giant for their obesity and related health issues. (They were the second lawsuit; the first was brought by Caesar Barbar in 2002, but withdrawn by his attorney Samuel Hirsch in favor of working with the younger plaintiffs Pelman and Bradley.) A *New York Times* article from February 3, 2003, said, "Just as Big Tobacco has been held liable for cancer, [plaintiffs' lawyers say] Big Food should pay for hypertension, diabetes, and heart disease. With obesity costing Americans an estimated $117 billion in 2000—and on its way, according to the surgeon general, to causing as much preventable disease and death as cigarettes — the damage awards could be enormous" (Cohen 2003).

As it turns out, they were not; the suit was dismissed, but with the ruling judge asking a question that has become increasingly relevant — and haunting — to health care providers everywhere: "Where should the line be drawn between an individual's own responsibility to take care of herself and society's responsibility to ensure others shield her? The complaint fails to allege the McDonald's products consumed by the plaintiffs were dangerous in any way other than that which was open and obvious to a reasonable consumer" (Wald 2003).

The third significant lawsuit involving fast food was *Monet Parham v. McDonald's Corporation,* in California in December 2010. It was dismissed by the presiding judge because, rather than seeing the Happy Meal and its accompanying toy as targeting children, he felt the issue was one of parental discipline and control, something that should not be decided in a courtroom (Andrews, February 2013).

While none of these, or myriad other, lawsuits resulted in damage awards, they have influenced the policies of fast food providers, who now post a calorie and ingredient poster, or provide such information in leaflets. Supersizing is also no longer a McDonald's option (thanks in large measure to independent filmmaker Morgan Spurlock's film by that name) and salads and fresh fruit have been added to menus.

Still, when New York City sought a legal ban on large soft drink sales, the effort failed, mostly because of its arbitrary enforcement. "The law would have restricted the sale of sugary drinks to no more than 16 ounces in restaurants, fast-food eateries, movie theaters and stadiums. But the law would have exempted a variety of retailers, including 7-Eleven, seller of the iconic 'Big Gulp' drinks, because it is regulated by the state, not the city" (Hicken 2013).

What does a failed New York City ban have to do with Appalachia? In rural Appalachian communities, populations tend to be low. In other words, such communities cannot support an Applebee's, a Trader Joe's, or any restaurant chain — or often mom-n-pop. Fast food franchises tend to be the only restaurants willing to locate in communities of 3,000 or less. Which means that, for better or for worse, fast food is eating out in rural Appalachia. There are only two choices: eat fast food, or eat at home. And while most people with health awareness will choose eating at home as often as possible, when it is not possible, they have a burger or chicken strips to look forward to.

What weight, if any, does this add to the question Judge Sweet asked back in 2003 echoes: where is that line between personal and societal responsibility? When it comes to corporate responsibility for products that harm health, such as sugary soft drinks, cigarettes and chewing tobacco, the question may still have no answer, but it has repercussions.

Before leaving this topic, an important distinction must be made between source accountability for products that could cause health harm if used to excess — which would include almost every substance under the sun — and those which can do nothing but harm, e.g., sodas and cigarettes. The public health community's need to pursue regulations on harm-only products is building, but this will be an uphill battle due to two main influences: powerful corporate lobbies with high economic stakes in the game; and an all-too-ready blame the victim mentality toward lower income and rural people.

Patient Responsibility in Diverse Populations

The second problem with the current use of patient responsibility in theory and policy is an unexamined, and, at times subtle, blame-the-victim mentality. Current policies, intervention plans, and by proxy the values structure of health care providers are largely based on what could be considered a fictitious homogenous standardization of any given population. "One key assumption informing health behavior theories is the standard or "norm" on which they are based: White, urban, middle-class Americans.... Until recently, leaders in the field of health behavior have been predominantly White, male, and middle class and employed at prestigious educational or research institutions" (Burke et al., 2009, p. 59S). As a result, theories and decisions about best practice have been based on research among

White, middle-class, young adults, the majority of them college students that formed a convenience sample population for academic researchers (Ajzen 1991; Emmons 2000). While effective for this particular population, such unexamined standardization has left lower income people, immigrants, rural populations, and those whose skin is not white without a voice — yet accountable for responsibilities they cannot, by definition, comply with. "Many of these [behavioral] theories end up blaming the victim for their own circumstances. 'What, you can't plan? What, you can't reason?' You know. 'You can't think? You can't believe? You don't have knowledge?...' We need to make explicit the assumptions that guide these theories and the limitations that underlie the theories" (Burke et al., 2009, p. 55S).

It is all too simple to turn non-compliance based on cultural differences or unexamined stereotypes into blame for those suffering health disparities because of them, and Appalachia has a history of such branding. Since the 1960s, when Appalachia and its poverty issues were "discovered" by President Kennedy's poverty tour, and publication of Jack Weller's *Yesterday's People*, and Harry Caudill's *Night Comes to the Cumberlands*, certain original labels have stuck. As early as 1965, health literature applied a few key stereotypes; Appalachians were lazy welfare recipients or job-to-job drifters; mistrustful of doctors and authority to the point of disregarding good advice; and fatalistic (Weller).

Consider the impact of assumptions such as this on clinical staff seeking to treat Appalachian patients. Blakeney did, in her career teaching students about Appalachian health needs. At her state-supported university within Appalachia, she found colleagues had excellent clinical skills and could break down complex ideas in clinical settings for the patient's care and for teaching students, but that "these health professionals often made very derogatory comments about the mountain people" describing them as "ignorant, uncooperative, difficult to manage, and unwilling to communicate. Their religious beliefs and family relationships were labeled as 'weird'" while patients were sometimes "discharged prematurely because some health professionals simply did not want to bother with people who 'weren't motivated to improve themselves'" (2005, p. 163).

In this milieu, a few interesting and subtle wheels within wheels begin to roll. The definition of personal responsibility hinges on the ability of a patient to not only understand, but act on, information provided with her best health interests at stake. Thus the patient's trust in the voice supplying this information must be solid. A patient who responds to a health care provider's command, "Jump off this cliff" by saying, "I think not" would never be considered irresponsible (although the provider might very well be). But what if a patient is told something so incongruous with her world-view that it sounds similar to "Jump"? What if she is informed that she needs immediate hospitalization and that her request to "have a day to pray about it" is "a nice thought but just wasting time you don't have?" What if a grandmother is told that the dinner she has enjoyed every Sunday since she can remember sitting at her own grandmother's table — ham, fried potatoes, green beans cooked in fatback, and a seasonal fruit cobbler, all accompanied with lard biscuits — is the reason she has Type II diabetes, and she must stop cooking it for her family? What happens when a sixty-five-year-old man is lectured by a twenty-something doctor about his nicotine habit? These are three different (and real) examples of the breaking of cultural taboos by which a doctor may never even know how insulting she has been to a patient: the first obviously denigrates a patient's spirituality, the second rudely yet subtly disdains the importance of family traditions, and the third disrespects elders in ways a young doctor may find entirely justified, while her patient may not.

While in each of these examples the doctor may have the correct information for her patient's personal health needs, the way in which the message is delivered must be culturally acceptable, or the message will fail. If it does fail, it may be counted as a breakdown of patient responsibility: the praying woman was called fatalistic and superstitious, the cooking grandmother considered not educated enough to grasp the consequences of her actions, and the elderly smoker refused to listen. But where does provider responsibility enter the equation? What if the doctor had said, "Here's my office; go in there and pray and I'll call you in half an hour." What if the grandmother had been referred to a nutritionist who said, "Let me show you how to make those great beans with liquid smoke instead, and did you know that Kroger's sells turkey ham?" What if the lecturing young doctor had recognized the age divide and asked her older nurse to deliver the news, or even approached with a gentle, "I recognize that you are my grandfather's age, so I am sorry if this seems like I am lecturing you..."?

In 2011 one of this paper's co-authors worked with an initiative out of the Virginia Department of Health's (VDH) Office of Rural and Minority Health, as it was then called. She traveled across rural Virginia seeking critical access hospitals (25 beds and smaller) that had or needed cultural competence in foreign languages. While talking with the dedicated staff— usually charge nurses or quality control specialists — she was struck again and again by the care and concern, not to mention the ingenious solutions, shown by nurses toward patients who had limited or no English language ability. Without denigration or annoyance, emergency room staff sought ways to fulfill their obligation to provide immediate care to those with life-threatening conditions — conditions that often could not be described by the patient or family members. Yet similar respect is, as Blakeney showed above, not always afforded rural Appalachians. One possible reason is the ingrained stereotypes that have existed for so long. But another has a difficult quagmire within it.

At a Cancer, Culture, Literacy conference in Florida in 2009, one of this paper's authors attended a debate about minority ethnicities and their undue burden of cancer. Someone brought up Appalachia's dismal cancer rates, and a Center for Disease Control (CDC) official said, "The problem with Appalachians is, they're white." No one else in the room reacted to this incongruous comment, and discussion moved on to African American needs in rural settings, not specifically Afrilachian. Afterward the co-author spoke with the man who had made the comment. He was an anthropologist working with the CDC's cultural competency measures, and he had more to say. "It's an ugly truth. No one wants to say so in a public paper, but since Appalachians are white, they're not seen as a vulnerable population" (private conversation).

In 2012, at the conclusion of the VDH project, the co-author was invited to present on Cultural Competency in Appalachia at the VDH's Rural Health Day, and suggested during the presentation that there was something incongruous about a region that had justifiably earned a reputation for racism, seeking the protection of minority status. A small ripple of laughter went through the audience, which was about 60 percent African American, 40 percent European American.

It is an odd, uncomfortable problem that vulnerable populations in America are not supposed to be White. Earlier this essay's research suggested that most policies were designed in favor of White as the norm. Appalachians, including those in urban areas, are about 84 percent White, 9 percent African American, 4 percent Hispanic, and 3 percent "other," mostly Native American. When one excludes cities, the White population jumps to an estimated 92 percent (ARC 2010 census data). And Appalachian White, as the CDC researcher hinted, is a few degrees off plumb from normal. Thus this majority within a minority area would benefit greatly from being declared a vulnerable population, one that requires particular cultural competencies from its health care deliverers.

This is not to say that other regions — the American Midwest, Cowboy Country, Northern Californians — do not also have their own cultures; of course they do. But the fact remains that where disparities reign among geographic populations of European descent, it is necessary to consider that area's cultural characteristics as needing special consideration. But this research focuses on rural Appalachians.

Cultural Competency's Effect on Personal Responsibility's Application

Cultural Competency is a term used in many capacities, but primarily intended to convey the idea that health care is delivered in specific geographic areas to people of particular mindsets. When working in areas that value specific traits or characteristics, it is important to recognize, respect and when appropriate harness these concepts as assets to providing care, rather than ignore or fight with them. As an example, people in southwest Virginia are considered (stereotyped, one could argue) to value their elders more than their urban counterparts or other European-American cultures. The ways in which older people expect respect from younger generations could come into play during clinical visits — and anecdotal evidence abounds that it has done so. When a younger medical professional lectures an older person about behaviors and choices the patient has made, the patient may evoke this cultural sense of elder privilege as a reason for disregarding the clinician's advice, or even leaving that clinic's care (Welch 2012). In order to provide effective care, the health professional must understand the expectations of polite versus rude behavior in any given culture. It may even be feasible to refer to cultural competency as part of the overall package of "provider responsibility" although this term would also include concepts such as HIPAA compliance and standards of care as well. These last two elements of provider responsibility are beyond the discussion boundaries of this paper; cultural competency as imbricated with patient responsibility will be its focus.

So if, in imparting information that is realistically in the best interest of an Appalachian patient's health (per the scenarios outlined above, e.g.) a doctor breaks a taboo, or appears rude, or seems uncaring because of a cultural faux paus, we can agree that this will negatively affect the patient's response to and belief in the information imparted. What if the doctor gets a further element of the culture wrong? What happens when a misunderstanding of specific challenges brought to the doctor's attention by the patient is ignored?

Perhaps the most poignant example of such ignoring comes from *Appalachian Women's Perceptions of Their Community's Health Threats,* an article famous among cultural competency workers for its use of focus groups and informants' own voices. In *Perceptions,* women lay much of the blame for the current prescription pain medication crisis of abuse in Kentucky at the feet of the region's medical providers.

Many of the women decried how physicians no longer spend time talking with patients and families, preferring instead to simply prescribe, in the words of 1 participant, "a quick fix." "There's a pill for everything. If you've got an ache, a twinge, a pain, just drive through the doctor's office and he'll write you something for a pill. I went to go get checked (for the flu) and the first thing — oh, here's you a pill. I don't want that. Just tell me what's wrong with me." ...

Throughout the focus groups, similar views were expressed about the substitution of prescriptions for caring, on professional, societal, and familial levels [Schoenberg et al., p. 78].

Medical providers in central Appalachia are sometimes noted to be quick with their prescription pads, yet slow to listen. In some cases, people object to pain medicine because they understand it is addictive; in others, they do not want the responsibility of something with a street value in their house, sometimes for painful reasons. In my family, a terminally ill member refused to take oxycodone home from the hospital with her, because her grandson "John" was physically stronger than her husband, and she knew "John" was in debt. She feared if she took the pills home, "John" would take them by force from the house, perhaps harming her or her husband in the process.

These are painful choices, but real ones. In a region with significant documentation of substance abuse, when a patient tells a doctor, "I do not want that," will a doctor listen to the underlying message, ask the right questions? Or will he assume ignorance and non-compliance and move on — perhaps having left a prescription slip behind?

Doctors are also perceived to prescribe medications the patient cannot pay for, dismissing requests for generics, ostensibly because the generics may not be as effective. However, one emergency room doctor in rural Appalachia recently spoke to this issue on condition of anonymity, and suggested that "too many of my colleagues are being taken to expensive lunches by drug companies" (private conversation).

The famed ethnographic field researcher Bruce Jackson once made the rather frustrated comment about fieldwork that, "I don't think you can ever fully know someone else's motives; you can only know for sure what they do.... Intentions, actions, and attitudes may have only coincidental relationships with one another" (1996). This is as true of doctor's motives as it is of patients. But the fact remains that responsibility for those actions is becoming an ever-increasing point of interest in how health care resources are allocated in the United States (Buyx 2008).

Analysis

Lest the arguments presented here be misconstrued, it is not the authors' contention that patient responsibility does not exist at all, but that it does not exist in a vacuum, any more than the social theories that formed or normed it as a concept exist in a sterile "all other elements being equal" environment. There are personal choices, but they are fewer and more contextually-influenced than one might think.

> Culture is not distinct from or equivalent to religion, politics, or any other social institution such as economics or kinship; rather, it is an integral part of all of them — forming them and being formed by them according to situation and circumstance. Thus, culture is a dynamic process that changes over time and across space, whether in contact with or in isolation from other groups, and is not a discrete entity with a material presence, fixed attributes, or clear boundaries. It is the outcome of the interactions, feelings, and thoughts of many people and their diverse, often overlapping, sometimes contradictory, attempts to make sense of their world and live in it. This view of culture differs from the discrete, bounded, identifiable categories taken up in social psychology (Triandis 1989) [Burke et al., 2009, p. 62S].

The classic definition of culture is acquired, learned patterns of behavior (Geertz 1973). Habits are formed by patterns of repeated behavior. Culture is patterns of behavior. It can be surprising how little idea people have that their own patterns of behavior are heavily informed by where they grew up, under what economic circumstances, and in what ethnicity.

This is the final examination of how cultural competency interacts with patient responsibility. When a habit is formed by culture — as in the case of the grandmother who grew up eating ham and biscuits on Sunday and began cooking it for her own extended family as the matriarch — it will be difficult to examine impartially. It will be as difficult for a cultural participant to separate habits from personal choices as is forcing recognition by a clinician of unexamined assumptions about patient behavior.

> In Bourdieu's theory of *habitus*, "unconscious" means an embodied awareness that influences practice yet is outside conscious awareness or below the threshold of consciousness. This is distinct from a psychological or Freudian concept of the unconscious or subconscious in that for Bourdieu, the unconscious is a product of social forces rather than individual psychology. *Habitus* exists only in and through the practices of individuals and their interaction with each other and their environment; thus, *habitus* "is not just *manifest* in behavior, it is an integral *part* of it (and vice versa)" [Jenkins 2002, p. 75, emphasis in original].

Habitus "shows that routine behavior is the product, not simply of biological or psychological motivation, but also of larger social, cultural, and historical forces. In doing so, it shows how individual behaviors relate to social rules and morality" (Crossley 2004, p. 239; Burke 2009, p. 63S).

Conclusion

Four main findings have resulted from this research:

1. Personal responsibility in large measure rests on unexamined assumptions of health theory and public health policy that privilege middle class urban white-skinned populations. The problematic nature of Appalachia as a white but rural population must be re-examined in this ongoing dialogue.

2. Elements of cultural competency and of provider responsibility to be competent to deliver a health message the patient can hear and respond to with self-efficacy is critical. Patient self-efficacy (based on having a choice, having been given information both understandable and useful enough to make it, and being competent in oneself to decide) is a large part of patient responsibility's definition.

3. The above is particularly important because of the increasing incorporation of personal responsibility into resource allocation, both at a federal or state policy level, and at individual caregiver levels "on the ground."

4. Corporate responsibility is currently a lighter piece of the dialogue surrounding patient responsibility; it must increase. Particular attention should surround corporations that manufacture items that have no positive health value (such as sodas or cigarettes).

Personal responsibility is destined to be even more of a buzzword in the public health lexicon than it has been to date, and it enters (re-enters?) a discussion edged by fears of limited resources, a fragmented care system, and national reforms touching on a hotbed of partisan politics. Whether its place will be based on an abdication of corporate responsibility, unexamined assumptions, and the dismissal of cultural competency in favor of one-size-fits-most policies and programs, remains to be seen. A mutual respect for patient and provider responsibility in an area rife with health disparity (such as southwest Virginia) would do much to decrease these disparities. It is in the best interest of public health officials to carefully examine previously unexamined assumptions surrounding patient responsibility in rural areas.

References

Ajzen, I. 1991. "The Theory of Planned Behavior." *Organizational Behavior and Human Decision Processes* 50: 179–211.

Andrews, Eve. 2013. "Justice for Big Food's Victims? Three Major Fast Food Lawsuits in the Past Decade." Food Tank, February 4, http://foodtank.org/news/2013/02/justice-for-big-foods-victims-three-major-fast-food-lawsuits-in-the-past-de (accessed 10 May 2013).

Appalachian Regional Commission. 2011. "Chapter 3: Race and Hispanic Origin." The Appalachian Region in 2010: A Census Data Overview. http://www.arc.gov/assets/research_reports/Chapter3AppalachianRegion2010-CensusReport.pdf (accessed 10 May 2013).

Bickelhaupt, D.L. 1974. "Rx for Rational Responsibility." *Journal of Risk & Insurance*, 41 (1): 1–8.

Blacksher, E. 2008. "Carrots and Sticks to Promote Healthy Behaviors: A Policy Update." *Hastings Center Report*, 38 (3): 13–16.

Boulding, K.E. 1972. "The Future of Personal Responsibility." *American Behavioral Scientist*, 15 (3), 329–359.

Brody, Jane. 2010. "You Don't Have to Smoke to Get Lung Cancer." *New York Times*. Retrieved from www.stltoday.com/lifestyles/health-med-fit/health/jane-brody/article_4870be4b-a379-554b-9d83-7c443b13f359.html (accessed 14 July 2010).

Brownell, K.D., Kersh, R., Ludwig, D.S., Post, R.C., Puhl, R.M., Schwartz, M.B., and Willett, W.C. 2010. "Personal Responsibility and Obesity: A Constructive Approach to a Controversial Issue." *Health Affairs*, 29 (3): 378–386.

Burke, N.J., Bird, J.A., Clark, M.A., Rakowski, W., Guerra, C., Barker, J.C., et al. 2009. "Social and Cultural Meanings of Self-efficacy." *Health Education & Behavior*, 36 (Suppl.1): 56S-81S.

Burke, N.J., Joseph, G., Pasick, R.J., and Barker, J.C. 2009. *Health Education & Behavior*, Vol. 36 (Suppl. 1; October): 55S-70S.

Buyx, A.M. 2008. "Personal Responsibility for Health as a Rationing Criterion: Why We Don't Like It and Why Maybe We Should." *Journal of Medical Ethics*, 34: 871–874.

Caudill, Harry. 1962. *Night Comes to the Cumberlands: A Biography of a Depressed Area.* Boston: Little, Brown.

Cohen, Adam. 2003. "The McNugget of Truth in the Lawsuits against Fast-Food Restaurants." *New York Times*, February 3, http://www.nytimes.com/2003/02/03/opinion/editorial-observer-mcnugget-truth-lawsuits-against-fast-food-restaurants.html (accessed 14 July 2013).

DeJong, W. 1993. "Obesity as a Characterological Stigma: The Issue of Responsibility and Judgments of Task Performance." *Psychological Reports*, 73 (3 Pt. 1): 963–970.

Emmons, K.M. 2000. "Health Behaviors in a Social Context." In L.F. Berkman and I. Kawachi (Eds.), *Social Epidemiology*, pp. 137–173. New York: Oxford University Press.

Frohlich, K.L., Corin, E., and Potvin, L. 2001. "A Theoretical Proposal for the Relationship between Context and Disease." *Sociology of Health & Illness*, 23 (6): 776–797.

Geertz, Clifford. 1973. *The Interpretation of Cultures*. New York: Basic Books.

H.R. Rep. No. 108-432. 2003.

Hermer, L.D. 2008. "Personal Responsibility: A Plausible Social Goal, But Not for Medicaid Reform." *Hastings Center Report*, 38 (3): 16–19.

Hicken, Melanie. 2013. "Judge Halts New York City Ban on Large Sugary Drinks." CNN *Money*, March 11, http://money.cnn.com/2013/03/11/news/companies/soda-ban/index.html (accessed 10 May 2013).

Kersh, R. 2009. "The Politics of Obesity: A Current Assessment and Look Ahead." *Milbank Quarterly*, 87 (1): 295–316.

Oxford English Dictionary. 2012. Oxford English online dictionary. Retrieved from http://oxforddictionaries.com/?region=us.

Puhl, R.M. and Heuer, C.A. 2010. "Obesity Stigma: Important Considerations for Public Health." *American Journal of Public Health*, 100 (6): 1019–1028.

Schmidt, H. 2009. "Just Health Responsibility." *Journal of Medical Ethics*, 35: 21–26.

Wald, Johnathan. 2003. "McDonald's Obesity Suit Tossed." CNN *Money*, January 22, http://money.cnn.com/2003/01/22/news/companies/mcdonalds/ (accessed 10 May 2013).

Weller, J. 1965. *Yesterday's People*. Lexington: University of Kentucky Press.

The Effects of Fatalism, Faith and Family Dynamics on Health Among Appalachian Youth

TAUNA GULLEY, RN

It is difficult to write about central Appalachia (the area often defined as West Virginia, southwest Virginia, northeast Tennessee, northwest North Carolina, and southeast Kentucky). There are many generalizations in the literature, yet great diversity lies within the region. While much of the region is rural, urban areas also exist.

Residents living in central Appalachia are not homogenous. Distinct economic classes and literacy levels show across the region. These socio-economic differences impact the health and wellbeing of the people who live there. Many rural Appalachian regions are still experiencing the long-term effects of poverty, unemployment, substance abuse, and illiteracy — problems whose negative effects on health are well-documented.

If it is difficult to write about Appalachians as a group without generalizing, it is exponentially harder to characterize Appalachian adolescents. Still, adolescents residing in rural central Appalachia do face many common challenges regarding the ability to develop healthy lifestyles, including cultural issues such as family connectedness and fatalism. In addition, healthy adolescent development requires the ability to develop a positive sense of self-esteem, and to feel self-efficacy; developing a healthy level of self-esteem and self-efficacy are important foundations for healthy functioning throughout life (Pender, Murdaugh and Parsons 2006). Unfortunately, some central Appalachian adolescents find themselves limited in their ability to develop healthy levels of self-esteem, due to several mitigating factors. These factors were explored in fieldwork I conducted recently in central Appalachia. The research found a few key factors that either created unexamined stereotypes, or created family dynamics that interfered with self-esteem development in adolescents, or both. We will examine each construct in turn.

Fatalism

Appalachians are often stereotyped as fatalistic, believing they have no control over their future. Fatalism has recently been defined as "the belief in a lack of personal power or control over destiny or fate" (Drew and Schoenberg 2011, 164). Self-efficacy, or the belief that one can do for oneself what is best for oneself in terms of choices and behavioral changes, is a more recent term used in health literature and related to fatalism, but its use began much later than the origins of fatalism in literature on Appalachia. The fatalism construct is used frequently in Appalachian literature, dating back to the 1930s, to describe factors influencing health behaviors and the decision-making processes of Appalachians.

In 1962, fatalism was defined as "the premise that life is governed by external forces over which humans have little or no control" when Thomas R. Ford conducted a survey of 1,466 Appalachian households from rural and urban areas (Ford 1962). Fatalism as a prevalent Appalachian value turned out not to be supported by Ford's survey data. He found that a large number of Appalachian residents relocated to other areas of the country in order to find better jobs and improve the economic situation for themselves and their families. Such action might be seen as contradicting the notion that Appalachians are fatalistic, without control over their own lives. In addition, survey results indicated Appalachian residents wanted their children to be high achievers in school and at work.

In 1968, Charles Valentine described Appalachian residents as fatalistic in his discussions about the culture of poverty model proposed by Oscar Lewis in 1961. The culture of poverty model suggested that all individuals living in poverty share certain beliefs and values, including a lack of planning for the future. Valentine compared Appalachians to "mainstream Americans" (middle class individuals who did not live in the Appalachian region). According to Valentine, Appalachians are fatalistic and believe they have no control over their future, while mainstream Americans believe they have control of their lives. In addition, Appalachians were described as impulsive, fundamental and individualistic while "mainstream Americans" were described as organized and rational (Valentine 1968). Odd as it may seem in the twenty-first century, this academic stereotyping went largely unexamined for two decades, until internal scholarship began to contest and counterbalance these external assumptions.

Appalachians tend to enjoy life at a comfortable pace. Returning to Lewis and his assertion that Appalachians were more "impulsive" than "mainstream Americans," impulsivity implies enjoying spontaneous activity, living for the moment, a present-oriented time perspective. Individuals who live in the present do not value scheduled activities; they do not adhere to time schedules or keep scheduled appointments. This live-for-the-moment orientation is not always conducive to health maintenance or health promotion efforts. When an individual lives in the present with little thought of the future, the individual cannot perceive the future benefit or detriment of today's actions.

That was the prevailing wisdom of 1976. Still, even recently the literature discusses fatalism in terms of time perspective. Time perspective can also be thought of as a unique way of thinking and acting based on a learned temporal focus, past, present or future. A majority of the literature on the subject is based on Phil Zimbardo's research on time perspective. According to Zimbardo and Boyd (2008) fatalism is an example of a present time perspective. Individuals who are fatalistic cannot connect today's actions with future consequences. Fatalists believe their behavior has no influence on future events. Individuals with a fatalistic perspective are not receptive to health promotion efforts. Additionally, fatalistic individuals have been linked to risky health behaviors.

For example, one study found that drug users who are predominantly present-fatalistic are more likely to share needles than individuals who are not fatalistic (Zimbardo and Boyd 2008). Little information exists in the literature regarding fatalism among adolescents in central Appalachia. Only one study was found that explored the construct fatalism among adolescents. Results indicated that Appalachian adolescents were more likely to be fatalistic than their non–Appalachian age mates (Phillips 2007).

Two main themes seem to affect perceptions of fatalism in central Appalachia. One is perhaps underexplored in academic literature. In the early 1900s, the coal industry positively impacted the economy of central Appalachia. However, in the last thirty years, a decrease in employment in the coal mining industry has resulted in worsening economic conditions for the region. Thus, in the central region, a reason people are viewed as fatalistic could be their dependency on a single extraction industry, and its slow, steady decline. Appalachians mine coal but rarely control its economic power, or their own. How does the long-term extraction of resources without investment in infrastructure affect the self-esteem, the self-efficacy, of the people who live in the region, who extract the resource, but who do not have long-term benefits from the same? Does disempowerment result in reduced self-efficacy, and thus fatalistic behavior?

Faith and Fatalism

A more common assessment is that individuals may assume a fatalistic time perspective as a result of religious beliefs. Welch (2011) discusses faith-based fatalism in *Self-Control, Fatalism and Health in Appalachia*. In that paper, faith-based fatalism, or the notion that "God will heal" may be detrimental to an individual needing specific medical intervention such as chemotherapy to treat cancer. However, as Welch (2011) pointed out, there are individuals who will follow all recommendations by physicians, while professing their faith in the healing power of God.

Smith and Denton (2005) state faith formation among adolescents is influenced by parental faith and expressions of faith. In other words, each generation learns from the generations above, most often from those in our own family. What we see and hear is generally what we grow up being and doing in our own lives. Findings from the *National Study on Youth and Religion*, a study examining the religious and spiritual lives of 3,290 teens, indicated adolescents thought faith was important; however, they could not state clearly how faith was integrated in their daily lives (Peters 2009).

Faith is an important aspect of Appalachian culture. When parents attend church regularly and routinely demonstrate expressions of faith such as praying, adolescents imitate this behavior. In this way, parental notions of faith-based fatalism pass from generation to generation. Faith fatalism describes individuals who believe their fate is pre-determined by the plan that God has for them.

Family Connectedness

Attachment to the community, family cohesion, and strong religious faith have also been identified as factors influencing health behaviors among Appalachian adults (Coyne, Demian-Popescu, and Friend 2006). The Appalachian region is known for its well-articulated history and diverse culture. Before Europeans came to the Appalachian region, the area was inhabited by Native Americans. Most of them were farmers and hunters. By 1761, most of the Indian lands were taken over by Europeans. After that, the Caucasian population in Appalachia grew rapidly.

Much of the Appalachian region's rural topography is farm land. Early inhabitants farmed the land and tended to have large families. The family was the center of life activities. Families had on average eight to fifteen children, who served as the labor force for the farm. Occasionally, it was necessary for families to join together for more difficult tasks such as building a house or a barn. Extended families became small communities. Together they celebrated happy occasions and mourned sad ones. As a result, the Appalachian culture is characterized by a strong sense of family and community. Even today, time spent with family in traditional events remains a defining characteristic of Appalachian culture.

The strong influence of family within the Appalachian culture plays a significant role in the health behaviors of the adolescents who live there. Many researchers have reported family connectedness as a protective factor against the initiation of negative health behaviors such as substance abuse, eating disorders, and early sexual activity (Viner et al., 2006). Family connectedness has also been associated with increased physical activity among adolescents. Sometimes this manifested in families finding ways to exercise together, or simply enjoy outdoor time in a recreational way, perhaps playing physical games such as touch football or baseball; but families with a closer dynamic also report better self-esteem and great self-efficacy, and thus better individual health choices among adolescents (Carter, McGee, Taylor and Williams 2006).

The family connectedness Carter et al. refer to is a healthy dynamic, but unfortunately familial influences can also work in quite the opposite direction. The following story is an example of a harmful situation told to me by a social worker:

> I was asked to do a drug screen on a lady whose child was in foster care. It was reported to us (social services) that she and her father were "shooting up" together. We obtained a drug screen on the female and sure enough, she was positive. I am not sure whether or not she was "shooting up" with her father; however, I do know this type of activity is a way of life for some people. They have been exposed to this type of activity (substance abuse) for so long they think it is normal.

How do we teach parents, children and adolescents the importance of encouraging positive connectedness among families is a means of promoting health. Unfortunately, the previous example illustrates the challenges that negatively affect the sense of family connectedness among Appalachian youth; other challenges include illiteracy and poverty.

The concept of family connectedness has been explored numerous times from various theoretical perspectives in order to gain an accurate understanding of the notion of connectedness within the family. Family connectedness is multifaceted and should be viewed from a theoretical perspective in order to be able to recognize the complexity of the concept. According to general systems theory, the notion of family includes the interactions with family members, other family systems and various environmental systems. From the perspective of general systems theory, family connectedness includes boundaries, communication, entropy, homeostasis, open and closed systems, feedback, purpose, relationship and wholeness (Becvar and Becvar 1982).

Family Connectedness and Boundaries

Boundaries within a family are defined by the patterns of behavior the value system will allow. Parent-adolescent boundaries should be clear and flexible. Flexible boundaries promote the development of identity, individuation and continuous connectedness within the family. When boundaries are violated, disconnect occurs. Unfortunately, in families where there is substance abuse, boundaries can become obscure to the adolescent and violation of boundaries is likely to occur.

For example, a parent who is a substance abuser will instill anxiety in the family system and eventually withdraw from the family. When this occurs, the adolescent loses the ability to please the parent. Then the adolescent will focus on personal desires which may disrupt boundaries and result in family conflict; the family becomes disconnected and the adolescent may become subdued and therefore incapable of developing an identity. When adolescents are unable to develop a self-identity, they become anxious, depressed, self-centered and exhibit decreased levels of self-confidence (Mayseless and Scharf 2009).

Boundaries within a family system promote healthy development for children and adolescents. Discipline helps to maintain boundaries within a family system. However, some parents do not know the proper way to discipline their children. According to one emergency room nurse:

> I just do not see much organized discipline in a lot of families with children and this is a big problem. We have parents who bring their child/children to the emergency room because the child acted out or may have gotten upset or angry at home and they want us to give them medications to calm the child down. Some parents even ask us to have their child committed to a state institution for behavioral issue.
>
> In addition, there are several families of single parent homes. The parent works hard to provide for the family and they feel if they discipline their children, they will not feel loved or they fear child protective services will take the child away from them. In contrast, we see parents who do not discipline because they just do not care what the child does or what happens to the child.

The advice a 92-year-old mother, grandmother and great-grandmother offered regarding effective discipline strategies was echoed many times in my fieldwork: "It will not hurt them to get a whipping; it will make them think more of you." However, this was balanced by opinions and comments such as, "I could not hurt them children," or "no one is going to hit my kids." These were common responses voiced by parents.

There are many debates about when and how to discipline children and adolescents. According to the American Academy of Pediatrics (1998) effective discipline requires the parent and child to have a loving supportive relationship. As a result, the child believes they are in a stable environment and they have a competent person taking care of them. In this way, parental responses have an impact on the child's behavior. The child wants to please the parent. As children grow into adolescents, parents must be flexible and willing to alter discipline strategies as the adolescent develops more responsible behavior.

Family Connectedness, Communication, and Entropy

Communication patterns define the nature of relationships within the family structure. For the adolescent, communication among family members must be open and honest, allowing the expression of ideas and experiences without fear of disapproval. Adolescents desire peer approval. They are frequently on Facebook or messaging their friends. One parent I interviewed spoke for many when she stated, "She won't tell me anything." Adolescents need time and space for their friendships and to develop an identity.

Entropy refers to disorder within a system. Adolescents need a structured environment to help lessen their struggle with role identity and personal autonomy. Substance abuse within a family system can result in disorder (a lack of structure and organization) within the system. Disorganization within a family system will result in disagreements among family members resulting in an abrasive emotional climate that is not supportive of healthy adolescent development.

Disconnected Dynamics

Increasingly in central Appalachia the buying, selling and trading of prescription drugs has resulted in a disconnect among family members. As a result, the foster care system has been flooded with children and adolescents needing foster home placement. As one social worker stated, "the caseload has increased substantially" due to the abuse of methamphetamines, prescription drugs and alcohol.

Ask any health care professional in central Appalachia, and they will confirm that the number of children in foster care is increasing. A majority of children in foster care are low functioning due to their home lives and past experiences. Many of the children growing up in foster care face developmental challenges such as separation anxiety from the parents and feelings of insecurity.

Stability and Connectedness

Homeostasis refers to any given system's ability to maintain stability. A family's ability to remain stable is dependent in the ability of its members to adapt to surrounding circumstances as time passes. When a child becomes an adolescent, parenting practices change in order to facilitate healthy growth and development for the adolescent. Parents of adolescents allow them more unsupervised time with friends and activities. Parenting practices associated with positive outcomes for adolescents are characterized by high-levels of warmth and moderate degrees of control (Lezin et al., 2004).

Open and closed systems refer to the boundaries a family creates among family members. Allowing the system to change gradually in response to input from other systems will enhance the health of the system. However, adolescents prefer a quick change in the family system in response to input from other systems. For example, John just got his driver's license, but his parents do not want him to drive on the interstate during the winter months, so John's driving is restricted to home, school and town. At Christmas time John's friends want to see a movie at the mall, and pressured by his friends, he drives to the mall. The family's ability to modify restrictions would accommodate John's desire to drive on the interstate. This decision requires flexibility and reasoning from parents so that John's need to develop independence and socialization can be facilitated.

Systems are goal oriented. The relationships among family members relate to the purpose of the system. Feedback serves to maintain stable functioning of the system in order to preserve its values and ensure the continued existence of the system. For example, if the adolescent in a particular family stayed out too late, feedback is required if this behavior is unacceptable within the family system.

Relationship refers to patterns of interactions among family members. From a systems perspective, individual family members are equal. The adolescent needs to feel equality within the family unit. When an adolescent feels equally powerful, willingness to openly share feelings and desires with family members which would enhance connectedness. Unfortunately, foster children report feeling insecure, helpless, anxious, and depressed (Lee and Whiting 2007).

Wholeness refers to the system being greater than the sum of its parts. Family members' interactions are not independent of the system; the behavior of one member can only be understood in the context of the family system. Stable family units encourage a healthy connectedness for its members. For the adolescent, implications for health interventions must be provided in the context of the family.

An example of an Appalachian family that exhibits a healthy sense of connectedness would include children who know their parent/caregiver cares about them and their feelings, listen to what they have to say and are interested in what goes on in their lives. In situations where these things are lacking, children feel disconnected which may result in anger issues or substance abuse in order to get attention. It is very important for parents to participate in the daily lives of their children in order for them to feel connected and have the ability to build close relationships with others.

Adolescents and Health Care

Emergency rooms have seen an increase in "cutters." A "cutter" is someone who cuts him or herself with a sharp object. Many adolescents cut themselves for attention, relief of stress or simply just because they can. They are trying to find something in their lives they can control. They feel powerless and perceive themselves in uncontrollable situations. Some adolescents see a lot of drug and alcohol use in their homes and homes of friends. Some reported witnessing verbal and physical abuse in their homes and neighborhoods.

Appalachians typically have a mistrust of healthcare workers (Simon 1987) and have traditionally used alternative medical treatments or home remedies for their ailments instead of seeking services from providers. For example, mineral oil has often been used for constipation, cod liver oil was used as a vitamin supplement. Cough syrup was made from moonshine and peppermint. Penny royal tea, otherwise known as "penny rile tea," was used for colds, the flu or an upset stomach. Rat's vein and goldenseal made a paste for poison ivy and aloe vera was used for burns. But what alternative medicine exists for a healthy family system?

Healthcare is a major concern for people living in Appalachia. Appalachian residents suffer greater health disparities than any other region in the United States. This is due to education levels, the lack of health insurance, and access to care. Due to the economic conditions, money is a factor determining care. One Emergency Room (ER) nurse stated:

> By coming in to the emergency room, adolescents will be seen and treated with or without money. There are no co-payments or money "up front" before being seen. Most doctors' offices require payment before seeing a patient who is uninsured. After the adolescent is seen and treated, they ask the ER staff to send the bill to their address. Emergency department visits are very expensive in comparison to other venues of care, i.e., the health department, outpatient clinic or physician's office. However, the majority of adolescents come to the Emergency Department without ever having been seen by a physician in an office or outpatient clinic. Either they do not have a family physician or have not attempted to get an appointment. Perhaps they do not realize they can be seen and treated at a local health department.

Another ER nurse said:

> We see a lot of adolescents in the emergency department. They come alone or with a friend, for treatment of various problems. Adolescents get very upset when the emergency department staff inform them they have to call their parent or guardian for permission to treat. Most teen girls know that they can be seen and treated for a pregnancy or pregnancy related issue. However, they do not realize if they come to be seen for bronchitis symptoms and are pregnant, the ED staff still has to contact a legal guardian for permission to see them and treat, because their complaint is not pregnancy related.
>
> Youth tend to feel overlooked, unimportant, and ignored. They come to the emergency department seeking attention. Many of the adolescents we see are sexually active, some as young as 12 years of age. We are seeing an increase in STDs [sexually transmitted diseases] and pregnancies, drug use/abuse, alcohol, and mental health issues, especially anxiety and depression.

Unfortunately, ER nurses are reporting an increasing number of adolescents brought to the emergency department because they have suicidal ideations. Someone, usually a parent, brings the adolescent to the ER for involuntary commitment. The parent states the adolescent is a risk to them self and the parent requests involuntary commitment for the adolescent. When this occurs, the medical provider will assess the situation and if it is deemed necessary, the individual is placed in a psychiatric facility for evaluation and treatment.

One nurse practitioner stated she frequently sees grandparents and great-grandparents bringing adolescents to primary care facilities seeking care for minor illnesses. The grandparent or great-grandparent has stepped into the role of parent usually because of prescription drug abuse. A huge issue with grandparents and great-grandparents acting as parent to an adolescent has been the disruption in school activities. In one instance I researched where an adolescent had to be placed with a great-grandparent, the adolescent had to stop participating in school activities. The grandparent was not healthy enough to provide the frequent transportation to and from school required for participation, which is unfortunate because participation in school activities is fun for adolescents and promotes positive development.

Conclusions

Appalachian youth have challenges that negatively impact their ability to develop healthy lifestyles, challenges that include substance abuse, illiteracy, high levels of unemployment and poverty. Disconnectedness with family members and a present fatalistic time perspective likely result in negative health behaviors and unfavorable social outcomes. When parents are unemployed, the family may be below the poverty level. In this case, the adolescent may not have the tools to develop a strong work ethic. When adolescents do not develop a strong work ethic, they may be unable to develop a sense of competence, the pride and joy of accomplishing a goal or a task. Lack of social competence results in feelings of insecurity, anxiety and decreased self-esteem.

Family connectedness promotes feelings of belonging. Feelings of belonging enhance self-efficacy, elevate self-esteem, promote a sense of security (Faircloth and Hamm 2005), and will be more likely to protect against health risk behaviors (Resnick et al., 1993). Self-efficacy is the ability to control future health and well-being which is inconsistent with present fatalism, the inability to control the future.

Fatalism is a time perspective, a learned characteristic that some believe can be modified. A present fatalistic time perspective can become more future-oriented by teaching adolescents to set reasonable short term and long term goals for themselves. The adolescent should regularly review and revise the goals. Making to-do-lists is another way to become more future-oriented. Even if family members may be somewhat fatalistic, adolescents should be encouraged to become more future-oriented. It is a healthier time perspective.

This paper has benefited from conversations with Renee Easter, RN; Dusta Loretha Boggs, RN, MSN, FNP; Kim Lawson; and others who wished to remain anonymous.

References

Bartkowski, John P., Xu, Xiaohe, and Fondren, Kristi M. 2011. "Faith, Family and Teen Dating: Examining the Effects of Personal and Household Religiosity on Adolescent Romantic Relationships." *Review of Religious Research* 52 (3): 248–265.

Carter, Melissa, Rob McGee, Barry Taylor, and Sheila Williams. 2006. Health outcomes in adolescence: Assosciations with family, friends and school engagement. *Journal of Adolescence*, Vol. 30, No. 1: 51–62.

Coyne, C.A., Demian-Popescu, C., and Friend, D. 2006. "Social and Cultural Factors Influencing Health in Southern West Virginia: A Qualitative Study." *Prev Chronic Dis*, 3 (4). http://www.cdc.gov/pcd/issues/2006/oct/06_0030.htm (accessed 10 January 2009).

Drew, E.M., and Schoenberg, N.E. 2011. "Deconstructing Fatalism: Ethnographic Perspectives on Women's Decision Making about Cancer Prevention and Treatment." *Medical Anthropology Q.* 25(2): 164–182.

Ford, Thomas R. 1962. The passing of provincialism. In *The Southern Appalachia Region: A Survey*, edited by Thomas R. Ford. Lexington: The University of Kentucky Press.

Huttlinger, K., Schaller-Ayers, J., and Lawson, T. 2004. "Health Care in Appalachia: A Population-based Approach." *Public Health Nursing* 21 (March/April): 103–110.

Lee, Robert E., and Whiting, Jason B. 2007. "Foster Children's Expressions of Ambiguous Loss." *The American Journal of Family Therapy* 35: 417–428.

Mayseless, Ofra, and Miri Scharf. 2009. Socioemotional characteristics of elementary school children identified as exhibiting social leadership qualities. *The Journal of Genetic Psychology*, Vol. 170, No. 1: 73–94.

Meyer, M.G., Toborg, M.A., Denham, S.A., and Mande, M.J. 2008. "Cultural Perspectives Concerning Adolescent Use of Tobacco and Alcohol in the Appalachian Mountain Region." *Journal of Rural Health* 24 (1): 67–74.

Pender, N., Murdaugh, C., and Parsons, M. 2006. "Stress Management and Health Promotion." In N. Pender, C. Murdaugh, and M. Parson, *Health Promotion in Nursing Practice* (5th ed.), pp. 201–220. Upper Saddle River, NJ: Prentice Hall.

Peters, Rebecca. 2009. "We Get Who We Are: Cultural Adult Faith Produces Cultural Adolescent Faith." *Christian Education Journal* Series 3, Vol. 6, No. 2: 376–383.

Phillips, Tommy M. 2007. Influence of Appalachian fatalism on adolescent identity processes. *Journal of Family & Consumer Sciences*, Vol. 99, No. 2:11–15.

Schetzina, K.E., Dalton, W.T., Lowe, E.F., Azzazy, N., von Werssowetz, K.M., Givens, C., and Stern, H.P. 2009. "Developing a Coordinated School Health Approach to Child Obesity Prevention in Rural Appalachia: Results of Focus Groups with Teachers, Parents, and Students [Electronic version]." *Rural and Remote Health* 9: 1157.

Simon, J.M. 1987. "Health Care of the Elderly in Appalachia." *Journal of Gerontology Nursing* 13 (7): 32–35.

Smith, C., and Denton, M.L. 2005. *Soul Searching: the Religious and Spiritual Lives of American Teenagers*. Oxford: Oxford University Press.

Valentine, Charles. 1968. *Culture and Poverty: Critique and Counter-proposals*. Chicago: University of Chicago Press.

Vincr, Russell M., Mary M. Haines, Jenny A. Head, Kam Bhui, Stephanie Taylor, Stephen A. Stansfield, Sheila Hillier, and Robert Booy. Variations in associations of health risk behaviors among ethnic minority early adolescents. *Journal of Adolescent Health*, Vol. 38 No. 1: 15–55.

Welch, Wendy. 2011. Self-Control, fatalism and health in Appalachia. *Journal of Appalachian Studies*, Vol. 17 No. 1/2: 108–122.

Zimbardo, Phillip, and John Boyd. 2008. *The Time Paradox: The New Psychology of Time That Will Change Your Life*. New York: Free Press.

Finding the Spark:
Enabling Community Participation
in Research, Planning and Delivery

TOM PLAUT

Reflecting on people working for social change, sociologist Richard Sennett has suggested that the power to change depends on credibility, which in turn depends on knowing "how to listen well" and engage with others, of "making *receptiveness* more important than *assertiveness*." His comments led to reflections on my own forty years of organizing and teaching in the Appalachian region and how academic agendas and perspectives have sometimes made us more assertive and less receptive to the cultural worlds and perspectives in the communities around us. Our assertiveness can and often has blunted our receptiveness. Sometimes we have assumed we "know" what's going on without first doing some common sense inquiry. Sometimes we have acted out of ignorance, to the detriment of research and projects.

Doing It Wrong

Some examples:

1. When we began public health organizing in Madison County, North Carolina, some Appalachian Studies Association colleagues voiced disapproval of our working with the local health department, whose staff, in their view, was anti–mountain culture/racist and "part of the problem." They had no experience with the department or its staff; they just assumed it was contrary to local ways of being and understanding. In fact, the health department director and staff were lifelong county residents.

2. When a Mars Hill College colleague and I attended a conference on the future of an Appalachian subregion, he was surprised to hear that a personal friend who was a planner for the county where the event occurred had not been invited. Either the campus-based organizers of the conference considered him "part of the problem," or they had never networked with local planning staff, thereby losing a valuable perspective and resource.

3. When we were assessing the potential of obtaining a 911 emergency response system in a mountain county, a fellow sociologist told me it was impossible. "You can't afford it," he said. "We studied this in the Regional Planning Council Health Services Committee and there is no way you can do it. Madison County hasn't the resources." Although this colleague was involved in Planning District committees, he had not networked locally and thus did not realize the resource potential for community action that eventually created a 911 emergency response system.

4. Mike, the executive director of a local health clinic, wanted the lawn mowed. A teenager had upped his prices and Mike told one of his van drivers to do it. The van driver refused, saying it was not in his job description and filed a grievance. After the Grievance Committee sided with the van driver, Mike left the clinic that evening only to find the driver mowing the lawn. "What are you doing?" he angrily asked. "Mowing the lawn," came the reply. "All you had to do was say we had a problem and ask if I'd help you. Just don't tell me what I've got to do." Mike learned that in mountain culture (and rural cultures in general) people value collaborative decision-making and resent any process that makes one person higher than another in status and authority (Hicks 1992).

5. Mary, a clinic receptionist and recognized community leader, was told by a visiting federal inspector she was not being professional when she greeted patients by their first name. "But I go to church with these people," she countered. "If I call them Mr. or Mrs. they'll think I've gone crazy. They'd ask me if I'd 'gone and got a big head.'" The inspector didn't appreciate the importance of personal, multi-stranded relations in everyday rural life.

I've made similar mistakes in assuming who should be part of a project. In the early 1970s, some sociology students and I researched and published (in a tabloid newspaper format) an analysis of housing stock in Randolph County, West Virginia. We printed some 200 copies and put them in markets and restaurants in Elkins, the county seat. It included a section about the dangers of mobile homes with aluminum wiring, which I assumed would incite the wrath of local realtors. However, a few weeks later a realtor stopped me in the street to say how much he had liked the paper. When I said I regretted that we couldn't print more of them, he asked why I hadn't asked him to help pay for the printing. It had never occurred to me to ask people whom I had considered "part of the problem" for help.

Another example: In 1972 my doctoral committee asked me to design and manage a public informational meeting on strip mining. With the help of a local Presbyterian minister, we held the meeting in the small mining community of Coalton. I remember very little about the event, except a feeling that we were talking when we should have been listening. The only community feedback was the antenna being broken off my car (not a very unobtrusive measure). Approval came from the minister and my dissertation committee back in the flatlands of Washington, D.C., but there was nothing from the pews; no connection had been made with the community.

A good measure of success in community research is what happens after a research project is completed. If research doesn't lead somewhere, why do it? Success may be more research, especially with community partners or practitioners or it may be projects, such as those described below in the Madison County, North Carolina, Community Health Consortium. The best descriptor here may be "sustainable." Academics often must contain field work within a semester or the parameters of a research grant. The challenge is to link a series of institutionally-limited projects to a broader vision. For some institutions it might be linking to public health initiatives, for others environmental concerns with local impact, such as mountain top removal in many Appalachian counties.

In my own career, the first real link between the college and the community began with a request to research the causes of conflict between local staff and patients and medical providers who had in-migrated from other parts of the country. One of those providers asked me to work with a young man dying of cancer in a remote hamlet on the North Carolina–Tennessee border and his family caregivers. This led to researching available services and systemic problems facing dying patients in our county and to training by an expert in the field named Elizabeth Kübler-Ross and subsequently more research that put me to work in the founding of the first hospice in western North Carolina in Asheville. Then came requests to talk about care for the dying in surrounding mountain counties and train people who established hospice programs in three of them. This work created the networking that led to work in other agencies, including the Mountain Area Health Education Center (MAHEC) in Asheville, Departments of Social Services, a Rape Crisis Center, school systems and juvenile justice programs. There was so much work that we created a special office at Mars

Hill College (CARA) to service research requests of agencies and organizations such as the Appalachian Sustainable Agriculture Project, which helps family farms grow and market their products. Over the years our work unfolded in the linking of our basic research capabilities to community needs in the context of multiple partnerships.

Doing It Right

In retrospect, my understanding and growing confidence in this process began back in West Virginia in the mid–1970s with a lesson in receptiveness that dramatically led to community mobilization and power. When I received a teaching appointment at a small liberal arts college, my wife, Marian, and I with our five kids moved to a small farm in a hamlet about 10 miles north of Elkins. It was a tightly-knit mountain community unused to newcomers, especially from the college, which at that time and place was reputed in some local churches to be a surefire path to Hell. Later we were told, upon our arrival, local folks said that "a professor from the college had bought Ike's farm to build an observatory on the hill to look at the moon." They got closer to the truth of who we were when we had to reach out to them to help us adjust to our new life on a hardscrabble hillside farm. As these neighbors learned about our family, they came to trust us and we shared knowledge on a range of subjects, from farming to child rearing.

Our five children attended a two-room school with three grades to a room, a pot-bellied coal stove and a kitchen in between them. Lunches were cooked by students' mothers. The bathrooms were his and her outhouses; outhouse tipping appeared to be an intramural sport. Our children and others from surrounding farms walked to Kerens School every day, having to negotiate the fast moving traffic on Route 219, especially lumber trucks. We had requested school zone warning lights, but were refused. A school board member in the county seat told me our "old time" school was an embarrassment to the county and the state and would be closed within a few years, when students would be bused to the "modern" consolidated facility ten miles away in the county seat.

Randolph County is a mountainous ridge and valley area of about 1,000 square miles, with a number of isolated communities. Many residents did not want their kids to be bused an hour or more to a school they did not know — or have any sense of control over, or any opportunity to participate in as parents. There was a deep, emotional split on the consolidation issue between those in the county seat and parents in outlying communities. Being a member of one of an outlying community, I had a pretty good sense of how these parents felt.

After the school board refused funding for lights, we asked if they could be installed if the community found the money. The answer was "yes," probably because board members believed that Kerens was poor and could never raise the $2,300 required. A few days later, a 15-year-old girl, riding a horse, was hit by a lumber truck at the school intersection. She was a friend of our kids and we knew her family well. Her mother and "Pop," the school maintenance person and a local farmer, had coached me through a nerve-wracking episode that required my reaching into a cow to assist the birth of her calf. Their knowledge had saved our milk cow's life.

The girl was thrown to the side of the road and bruised, but not seriously injured. The neighborhood gathered at the family's house, which was close to the intersection where the accident had happened. We discussed how to overcome the resistance of the school board. I brought journalism skills to the meeting, having been a reporter for the *Baltimore Sun*, and so I wrote a press release. We also decided to have some of the children go on the local radio to ask families in the county to "just send a dollar for 'The Kerens Lights for Life Campaign.'" In doing so, we hit a nerve in county politics and the spark for action. We received close to $3,000 within a week and the county newspaper ran several articles on the story. (Some school board members, offended by the challenge to their authority by a small, rural and poor community, went to the president of Davis and Elkins College with a request that I be fired.)

The Lights for Life Campaign honed a template for social research/ action research that has served me well in the ensuing years:

1. Start by listening, not talking
2. Let the community decide when you understand what the issues are. (Even if you think you "get it," for collaboration, community members have to agree.)
3. Help the community define what it can do
4. Locate the energy and passion that can engender the "political will" for action
5. Help clarify goals and objectives
6. Offer whatever skills you (and your students) might have to facilitate the process

This process is the core of Community Oriented Primary Care (COPC), which I learned about after moving to Madison County outside of Asheville, North Carolina, in the 1970s. In 1988, I was asked to work on a community-based health program grant proposal to the W.K. Kellogg Foundation which was funded in July 1989. We based resulting Madison Community Health Project on the COPC model, which involves an assessment of the health strength and needs of the population of a defined geographic area. The definition of "community" is at the core of COPC theory and practice. The community, not "outside experts," such as medical providers or other professionals, defines its own needs and realities. The community — in dialogue with medical and human services professionals — consequently plays a major role in determining health-related interventions. If the professionals take too strong a leadership role, they lose the community support and the interventions fail or their impact is greatly reduced (Maguire 1987; Cancian and Armstead 1990; Shaler 1992).

COPC was conceived by two physicians, Sidney and Emily Kark, while working among the Zulu in South Africa in the 1940s. They defined a four stage process:

1. Defining the community — meaning the total population in a geographic area, not just users of the medical center. Studying the community, including its social institutions, structure and patterns of relationships, traditional healing methods, diet and economy.
2. Identifying community understandings of health problems and healing practices.
3. Involving the community in determining priorities in health needs and designing and implementing appropriate health interventions.
4. Ongoing monitoring of projects to evaluate their effectiveness and enable their ongoing modification (Kark 1981; Nutting 1990; Trostle 1986).

But what does "community" mean? COPC required (and the lessons learned in Kerens reminded me) that we ask Madison County residents for their own definition. The Kellogg Foundation and the grant writers had assumed the county was the community. But local informants disagreed, providing us with a maze of distinct kinship-based clusters of families determined by 19th century settlement patterns in a county containing some 430 square miles of mountainous terrain along the North Carolina–Tennessee border. To clarify conflicting definitions, we asked the county's three postmasters to work with their mail carriers to map communities within their zip code areas. Their maps were refined in discussions with local informants. A total of 72 units were identified, along with 350 "community helpers" (defined as people whom residents of a specific community would call if they needed advice or assistance). Thus, many residents did not see the county, but the traditional, kinship-based neighborhood of the mountain "cove" as "their community" (Eller 1982).

Three months of listening enabled us to draw a map of resident-defined communities, which ended up hanging in the county's Board of Elections office. Furthermore, we learned that some of these communities got along with each other, while some saw others as competitors and a few had grudges going back to the Civil War. The mapping exercise emphasized the project should not plan for "community organization" because there were plenty of communities already well organized in frameworks comfortable for their residents. The challenge for the project was to find issues that could bridge over community differences to create a county-wide basis for action. How could we find such issues?

In the fall of 1989 we conducted 40 "natural" focus groups across the county: 14 with community groups; seven with teachers; eight with social services, mental health and community support personnel (the sheriff's office, Extension Service, day care and congregate meal site staff); and 11 with medical providers. "Natural" focus groups are those in which participants already know each other through work or community life. Traditional focus group methods require participants share specific characteristics, such as residential type, or income or educational levels, but that they should not be acquainted with each other (Morgan 1993).

The setting for each focus group was its own turf, be it a school, a fire department garage, a church or an office. Field notes from an evening session with a Volunteer Fire Department indicate the kind of data that is only accessible through this natural focus group approach. The men were uncomfortable and annoyed at being asked to talk about problems in health and health care services delivery. Farmers, factory workers and small businessmen, they were not accustomed to being asked for their insights and opinions. Our notes report the session "started with silence," finally broken by soft-spoken, apologetic statements:

"We're really not the ones to ask about this."

"Basically, we're a pretty healthy county."

It took almost an hour for a sufficient level of trust to develop. Once they came to believe that we really were there to listen (and not impose our views or agenda on them), the men seemingly gave each other permission to talk honestly. An ambulance driver started the discussion by sharing an incident:

> One time a man died of a heart attack and we waited three hours for authorization to move the body. His grandchildren kept on coming in the bedroom and asking "why is grandpa lying there" ... "why won't he come out and watch TV with us?"

The group felt that the story of the grandfather's death exemplified a pattern in relations between county doctors, who served as medical examiners, and themselves. Participants recounted a series of incidents indicating their frustration with physicians whom they felt held them in low esteem:

- "The boy's body lay in a ditch for three hours before a medical examiner [a job held by local physicians] would let us move him."
- "It took an hour and forty five minutes for a medical examiner to move K's body to the funeral home. We had to sit there and watch the 'ooh-ahh crowd' stand there and stare at the body."
- "The doctors don't take any pride in helping the ambulance service in a wreck. The doctor charged me $35 and then told me 'you have to stay out of the dust for a while.' I'm a farmer. How am I going to stay out of the dust?"

As the group process developed, participants moved from sharing information to expressions of frustration, anger and resentment at, in their view, not being considered equal partners with other providers in medical emergencies. This is a continuing problem between medical providers and emergency responders. When a friend collapsed at a Christmas concert in 2012, an EMT arrived only to have his blood pressure cuff taken out of his hands by a woman who announced, "I'm a physician." After several minutes of her not being able to get a blood pressure reading, the EMT said, "It's my equipment. Please let me use it." He got the reading and my friend was rushed to an emergency room. The taking of his equipment by a person who took her superior status for granted is something emergency responders commonly experience and find unnecessary and humiliating.

Towards the end of the session, one participant, his chair tilted back against the cinderblock garage wall and a baseball cap pulled low over his eyes, broke his evening-long silence with a summary: "Look, just tell 'em that we're plain tired of being shit on."

When asked what might be done to improve the medical services, one respondent evoked cheers from his fellows by suggesting we nail the doctors' "feet to the floor and burn the building!" His cathartic response led to further reflections of the men's place in a county suffering the demise of farming and loss of its limited industrial base, while an increase in services brought in new kinds of people with different lifestyles and value systems. The doctors were described as "not what we're accustomed to."

- "They've hired hippies. They don't dress right."
- "That P.A.— he never takes a bath." (This comment was a real challenge for the assistant moderator that night, who happened to be the

P.A.'s wife. She was very cool and composed, containing her protestations until we were back in the car.)

- "They're strange. They're different. You go to the market and see a strange looking person and you say 'oh, that must be one of our doctors.'"

We found frustration across the groups. Among the teachers' comments were

- "What do you mean 'how do I know my students have dental problems?' I look in their mouths! One child continually pulls his lip down to hide the whole in his front tooth."
- "Many kids are so sick from the school bus ride [on twisting mountain roads] that we have them put their heads down on the desk and rest for the first period."

Misinformation and distrust between agencies led us to hold an "agency fair" in a community college, enabling each agency to tell the others' staff what they did. It proved to be an important step in fostering interagency collaboration in future projects, especially in grant writing.

We also provided feedback to the medical providers. Some were surprised and offended, when I said beards made many clients uncomfortable. One, who later asked me to advise her daughter on an academic project and is now the pediatrician for my grandchildren, accused me at the time of "stirring up the county against us." But these providers, in the main, were willing to change to accommodate patient perceptions. (In later trainings with other groups, I found medical providers with little respect for their patients. A urologist commented in a COPC workshop, "Why should I listen to someone who can't afford my services?" There have been derogatory comments about Appalachian people, alleged incest and bizarre faith traditions by professionals well trained in their specializations, but who have little cultural awareness or sensitivity.)

As the COPC work in Madison County continued, the focus groups and discussions with local leaders developed enough common ground to begin a series of initiatives in the winter of 1990, with across-the-county involvement and support through the focus group–generated "Madison Community Health Project Community Advisory Board," which became known as "The CAB." The CAB grew out of a few citizens and county agency staff who had been involved in the proposal writing sessions that had procured the W.K. Kellogg Foundation funding of the health project. In the first two years of the project, the CAB grew from 25 to 40 people representing most county public and private service agencies as well as community groups.

The first CAB project actions were non-controversial:

- An oral health/dental sealant program for school children
- Annual health fairs for seniors reaching over 500 people each year
- Support for parents of newborn children in a pilot school district by specially trained lay volunteer women selected by the PTA, which had been found to be a strong and high-functioning local grassroots organization
- Forums for high school seniors on AIDS, stress and stress management
- Flu and pneumonia vaccinations for people over 65
- A newspaper column on health issues, written on a rotating basis by CAB members
- Publication of two resources guides, one for parents and a second for the elderly
- Co-sponsorship of forums on national health care and insurance reform

The 40 focus groups also told us to avoid the "hot-button" issues of tobacco cessation, family violence and alcohol abuse. These issues would have divided medical, social services providers and teachers from community groups at the start of the project, but could be addressed at a later time after sufficient trust had been generated between groups.

In September 1992, the CAB scored a major success (and proved the academic naysayers wrong), when it won a $220,000 competitive grant from the U.S. Department of Health and Human Services. The grant financed a 911 emergency telephone system (which replaced the 13 different emergency numbers) and provided emergency and injury prevention training for county residents. The grant not only funded important and needed services, but made a clear statement to the people (whose anger and frustration was manifested in the group interviews at the start of the project in 1989) that their concerns had been heard and had sufficient impact to win a competitive national grant (only 27 awards were given among 260 applicants). A year later the CAB won an additional $270,000 to further develop the emergency response system. Volunteer fire departments and other community organizations, assisted by college students, saved thousands of grant dollars by undertaking the mapping and street renaming required to make the 911 system work.

By 1993 the CAB had become the "Madison Community Health Consortium" and a national model for grassroots community health initiatives. The Kellogg Foundation provided funds for its members to conduct training in other counties and states. And other funding sources took notice. In 1995, we received a $175,000 grant for a two-year Diabetes and Nutritional Counseling Education Program. The trust between agencies and flexibility in work patterns was demonstrated when the grant writing team was able to change the designated recipient of the funding from the county health department to the private medical program without any fights over "turf." By this point in trust building, key players were able to comfortably work for the common good of the county rather than the benefit of their individual agency.

When a film crew interviewed the health department director about the impact of the consortium, she replied:

> It's probably the best thing that ever happened to Madison County — the best thing that's ever happened to the health of the people of Madison County. We have had an impact on just about every segment of the population. We have taken on projects that impacted health needs that were identified by the community. That's where it starts and that's the only way you're going to make a difference.

Students Serving Community Projects

Regional Studies faculty and students at Mars Hill College benefited from the Consortium's research and action. We supported community challenges to proposed research methods, namely don't do surveys, rather go into the communities and talk to residents on their own turf; in this instance qualitative methods trump the quantitative. Emphasize community strengths — map for assets, not weaknesses.

The CAB projects enabled students to gain field experience in data collection, analysis and feedback to the community. They were able to begin assembling their own "toolboxes" of research skills, which have served them well in later graduate work and employment.

In the early 1990s, we were invited to partner on a summer project with an agency in the coal fields of Kentucky, assisting their community assessment. Our first meeting with our clients, who were local women, began with their venting deep resentment about previous college groups. They saw those college groups as coming with their own agendas and preconceptions of mountain people, what their capabilities were and that they weren't smart enough to understand. The anger of these women ran deep, so deep they were not sure they wanted to work with us. Given their feelings, I was surprised that we had been assigned to work with them. I had been led to believe we were responding to a community's request, but it turned out that the women had felt they could not turn down a university consortium's request to be a field site. The atmosphere improved only when I said words to the effect of "when you call a plumber, you know what you want fixed and she or he will know how to do it. Just think of us as 'data plumbers.' Tell us what you want to know and, using our tools (SPSS, Word and Excel and the skills required to use them), we'll help you find the answers." Once they began calling me "Tom the Plumber" we were able to start the project.

For students to participate in this community-directed research, they had to have a genuine respect for local people and proficiency in skills for the job. They had to be ready to work as apprentice data plumbers. For the Whitely County project, my students brought a working knowledge of how to gather and interpret quantitative data. They were reasonably proficient in basic data entry and analysis. They knew the basics of the SPSS statistical package. Much of is this is mechanical, so they had to be mechanics. Once they had the data in hand, they could reflect on their meaning, as enriched by the stories and other qualitative insights of the community women. It was a good summer project with a final product for the agency and a good training experience for students. This project emphasized that success in community-campus partnerships depends on teachers and students need to enter the field with well-defined skills with trust and respect for clients.

CARA: A Program for Training Students in Field-Ready Proficiency

At Mars Hill, many students developed a field-ready proficiency through experiential training at CARA, the Center for Assessment and Research Alliances. "Research alliances" meant just that: projects developed in concert with groups and agencies, such as the Appalachian Sustainable Agriculture Project, the Mountain Area Health Education Center in Asheville, victim assistance and juvenile justice programs, a genetics center, school systems and health and social services departments across the mountain counties of Western North Carolina.

CARA grew out of senior seminar research projects which generated requests for help in needs assessment and program evaluation. A break came with my being named assessment officer for the Kellogg Foundation–funded program mentioned above. Focus groups and other research provided opportunities for students. From the Kellogg Foundation project on, we were flooded with requests for help. Whenever possible, we connected community research to classes. By the mid–1990s, we had too many student researchers disrupting life in the Social Sciences building, so the college provided separate office space in another building. When classes could no longer cover research requests, we recruited students and paid them. CARA brought in enough contract income to cover much of our salaries and expenses, thereby becoming a partially self-supporting laboratory for the social sciences. (We were never successful in arguing that the college administration should include CARA in the budget just as it did with Natural Sciences laboratories.)

Students were trained through four levels of competence:

1. An introductory period involving supervised quantitative data entry and cleaning
2. Individual responsibility for data entry and cleaning for projects
3. Data analysis, introduction to qualitative techniques and report writing
4. Project and survey design and management, including negotiating contracts

The students who had the drive to work through these stages were able to use their training and research publications at Mars Hill for employment or graduate school. Virtually all the students who worked through the third stage found they were able to gain admission to graduate programs or find jobs using the quantitative and qualitative research skills they learned in our center.

One graduate did data analysis for a hospital before going on to graduate school. Today she has a PhD and is deputy director of a memory clinic in a university hospital. Another did a stint in the Peace Corps in Niger before entering a doctoral program in International and Women's Studies at Brandeis. At the time of this writing she has returned to Africa to do field work. Another CARA alumnus received Master's degrees in urban planning and public administration from UNC Chapel Hill before going to work in a municipal planning department. Another is teaching at the University of Kentucky, having completed his doctorate in Blacksburg, Virginia. Another became a consultant in research design and SPSS for East Carolina University faculty and staff.

These students are unique in that in addition to classroom learning they *learned by doing* tasks over and over again in CARA. They learned as apprentices in trades have done for centuries, working alongside journeymen in contracted field research. One psychology major told a visiting team from the universities of California and Michigan that she had "learned much more here (in CARA) than I have in my research classes." The concrete experiences in a clearly visible progression of skill levels gave students the confidence to decide when they were ready to move ahead to the next skill level. The ability to monitor and measure their own progress helped students better understand their personal learning styles and, at the same time, demystify academia.

CARA still exists almost a decade after my retirement, although currently in reduced form. The structure of a liberal arts program seems to be at odds with a skills-oriented, experiential training program in social research. It should not be. The social sciences need to respond to the growing concerns over the costs of higher education and the need to link education with employment markets by assuring their graduates have concrete skills for the trade. The fact that skill sets are evolving continually in this era of rapidly changing software is no excuse for our not providing students with a workable toolbox of skills. The often-cited need to train students to be flexible and creative does not preclude providing them a toolbox for whatever comes after graduation.

CARA has not single-handedly caused social change, but it has partnered with community groups and agencies to do so, often in ways that are off the academic radar. The Appalachian Sustainable Agriculture Program, the Madison Community Health Consortium, the Hot Springs Health Program, Project Phoenix (substance abuse prevention and counseling), hospices, school systems and other community-based programs continue to provide their services, often refined by community feedback. It is evidence of the sustainability in this approach to community partnering, networking and research. CARA also generated tens of thousands of dollars in income for Mars Hill College.

Returning to Richard Sennett's point about listening and receptiveness versus talking and advocacy, I believe we need to be more deliberate in training people to do the former. Valuing listening/inquiry over lecturing/telling is a shift in what many teachers and other professionals do, but I have come to prefer Tom the Plumber over Dr. Plaut. The continuing success of our CARA-affiliated graduates argues for college and university training programs that teach and model:

1. Ongoing relationships with local organizations and agencies needing assistance in research and evaluation. These relationships make real world research experience possible at the undergraduate level.
2. Research in adequately equipped laboratories. (If institutions fund natural science laboratories with microscopes and Bunsen Burners, they should also fund social science laboratories with computers and appropriate software. SPSS has proved adequate in doing and teaching quantitative research.)

3. Specific research skill sets. CARA required competence in
   a. SPSS for
      i. Data entry
      ii. Data aggregation
      iii. Basic data analysis
   b. Interviewing methods — how to listen
      i. Individual interviews
      ii. Groups and focus group sessions
4. Clear and concise writing up of results
5. Survey development and administration
6. Project proposal design and budgeting
7. Presentation of research results
   a. In academic settings
   b. In community settings, the importance of using community members in explicating results

There are professionals in any field who "know they know," which is an assumption that can cloud their assessment as they move into a project. Others, curious and often excited by the challenges of discovery, enter a situation first by listening. I began this paper with examples of colleagues who, based on their definitions the world, *knew* I couldn't trust or work with the staff of a health department or a local planning department. They were wrong on both counts. Experience suggests that inquiry is best for entry into community-based and partnered research. The discovery of community definitions of things like health, healing and community leads to collaborative research and sustainable solutions.

References

Cancian, Francesca M., and Cathleen Armstead. 1990. "Participatory Research: An Introduction." Paper presented at the American Sociological Association Convention, Washington D.C. August.

Hicks, George. 1992. *Appalachian Valley.* Long Grove, IL: Waveland Press.

Kark, Sidney. 1981. *Community-Oriented Primary Health Care.* New York: Appleton-Century-Crofts.

Maguire, Patricia. 1987. *Doing Participatory Research: A Feminist Approach.* Amherst, MA: The Center for International Education, School of Education, University of Massachusetts.

Morgan, David L., ed. 1993. *Successful Focus Groups: Advancing the State of the Art.* Newbury Park, CA: Sage.

Nutting, Paul. 1990. *Community-Oriented Primary Care: From Principle to Practice.* Albuquerque: University of New Mexico Press.

Plaut, Thomas, Landis, Suzanne, and Trevor, June. 1992. "Enhancing Participatory Research with the Community Oriented Primary Care Model." *The American Sociologist* 23, 4.

Plaut, Thomas, Landis, Suzanne, and Trevor, June. 1993. "Focus Groups and Community Mobilization: A Case Study from Rural North Carolina. In David L. Morgan, ed., *Successful Focus Groups: Advancing the State of the Art.* Newbury Park, CA: Sage.

Sennett, Richard, "A Credible Left." *The Nation*. August 1–8, 2011.

Shaler, George. 1991. "An Assessment of the Madison County Community Oriented Primary Care Project's Community Advisory Board." Chapel Hill: Health Behavior & Health Education Department of the University of North Carolina

Shaler, George. 1992. "Putting the Community Back in COPC — The Madison Community Health Project." A Master's Paper in the Department of Health Behavior and Health Education, The University of North Carolina at Chapel Hill.

Trostle, James. 1986. "Anthropology and Epidemiology in the Twentieth Century: A Selective History of the Collaborative Projects and Theoretical Affinities." In Craig R. Janes et al., eds., *Anthropology and Epidemiology*. Boston: D. Reidel.

About the Contributors

Mark **Dignan**, PhD, MPH, is a professor in the Department of Internal Medicine and director of the Prevention Research Center at the University of Kentucky. His research focuses on community-based cancer prevention and control, including reducing health disparities among Appalachian populations. These include projects on diabetes, colorectal cancer screening, adherence with follow-up for cervical cancer and energy balance.

Gretchen E. **Ely**, PhD, MSW, is an associate professor at the University of Kentucky, College of Social Work. She earned a doctorate from the University of Tennessee and a master's degree from Washington University in St. Louis. Her research is focused on women's health disparities and health access.

Morgan **Fields** is a PhD candidate in social work at the University of Louisville (anticipated graduation 2015). She received a MSW from the University of Kentucky.

Bob **Franko** works at Cherokee Health Systems in Knoxville, Tennessee, and has been employed in the healthcare safety net system since 1996. He received both his undergraduate and graduate degrees from Purdue University. He works with clinics all over the country on better integrating their primary care and behavioral health services.

Carl J. **Greever**, MD, is a graduate of West Virginia University and the Medical College of Virginia. A charter diplomate of the American Board of Family Medicine, he practiced family medicine in Appalachia for five decades. He also served as health commissioner of the Jackson County (Ohio) Health Department for three decades.

Tauna **Gulley** is an assistant professor of nursing at the University of Virginia's College at Wise. Her dissertation research focused on fatalism and the physical activity behaviors among central Appalachian adolescents.

Sue Ella **Kobak** is a native east Kentuckian who has lived in Lee County, Virginia, for nearly three decades with her husband, Dr. Art Van Zee. She acts as a community organizer, seeing her role in a community as a responsibility to organize around problems and needs of that community.

Tony **Lawson** lives in Millers Chapel, a rural community in Lee County, Virginia. He directs the PACE plan at Mountain Empire Older Citizens, Inc. Previously, he was with the Graduate Medical Education Consortium at UVA's College at Wise and Stone Mountain Health Services, a network of health centers in southwest Virginia.

Marilyn Pace **Maxwell,** executive director emeritus of Mountain Empire Older Citizens, Inc., earned a BS from the University of Alabama, an MSW from the University of North Carolina and a post-master's certificate in aging from the University of Michigan Institute for Gerontology. She is a forty-year veteran of asset-based community development work in central Appalachia.

Steve **North,** MD, MPH, is a family physician and adolescent medicine specialist in Mitchell County, North Carolina. He is the founder of the MY Health-e-Schools school-based telemedicine program that provides access to care for 4,000 students at 14 schools in the Blue Ridge Mountains of western North Carolina. He also serves as the medical director for outpatient telehealth for the Mission Health System.

Tom **Plaut** taught sociology in Appalachian colleges from 1972 to 2005. He conducted research and training for health departments and the Mountain Area Health Education Center (MAHEC) in Asheville, especially in the development of county-based public health partnerships. Before his retirement he directed the Center for Assessment and Research Alliances at Mars Hill University. He continues to provide training at MAHEC and area universities.

A. Carole **Pratt** practiced general dentistry for 32 years in rural Virginia, was a National Rural Health Association fellow during health care reform, and more recently was a Robert Wood Johnson Foundation health policy fellow serving in the Washington office of Senator John D. Rockefeller IV. She is a consultant for the proposed dental school at Bluefield College in the Central Appalachians.

Sarah **Raskin**, MPH, is a PhD candidate in medical anthropology at the University of Arizona. Her dissertation is an ethnographic exploration of oral health and dental care in far southwest Virginia, which is her childhood home. Research interests include critical public health, representations of illness, structural interventions and the politics of rurality.

Esther **Thatcher** is a PhD candidate at the University of Virginia School of Nursing, where she is researching healthy food access in rural Appalachia. She earned a degree in rural sociology from the University of Wisconsin–Madison, and has worked in community health in Latin America as well as Virginia.

Rachel **Ward** is a doctoral candidate in public health at East Tennessee State University, where she researches the intersection of local agriculture and public health. She has an MPH from East Carolina University and a bachelor's in public policy analysis from the University of North Carolina.

Wendy **Welch**, MPH, PhD, is the executive director of the Graduate Medical Education Consortium and Area Health Education Center of Southwest Virginia. She is the author of *The Little Bookstore of Big Stone Gap*, a memoir about the bookstore she and her husband run and the community that surrounds it.

Christian L. **Williams,** MPH, is a DPH candidate in the Department of Community and Behavioral Health at East Tennessee State University. She serves as the academic health department coordinator for Sullivan County Health Department in Blountville, Tennessee. She worked as a research assistant on *Team Up for Healthy Living*, a peer-based intervention focusing on reducing adolescent obesity in southern Appalachia.

Index

Page numbers in **bold** *italics* indicate pages with figures and tables.

CPSIA information can be obtained
at www.ICGtesting.com
Printed in the USA
LVHW091546190720
661081LV00005B/1601